LOW FODMAP AI COOKBOOK FOR BEGINNERS

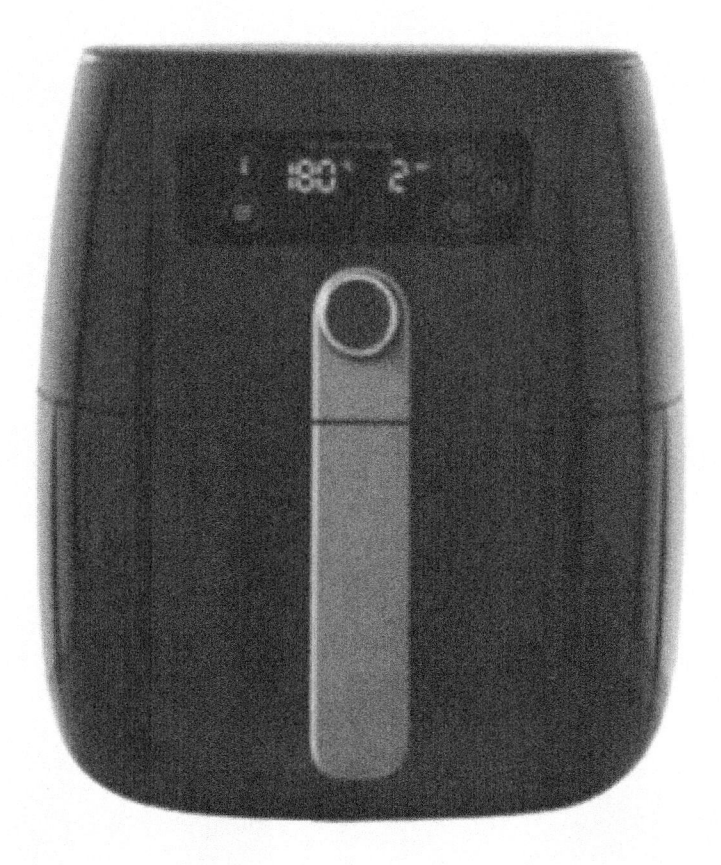

The Comprehensive Guide to Cooking Delicious and Nutritious Low Fodmap Recipes with an Air Fryer

Anne J. Henderson

All rights reserved. No part of this publication may be reproduced, distributed, or transmitted in any form or by any means, including photocopying, recording, or other electronic or mechanical methods, without the prior written permission of the publisher, except in the case of brief quotations embodied in critical reviews and certain other noncommercial uses permitted by copyright law.

Copyright © (Anne J. Henderson), (2023).

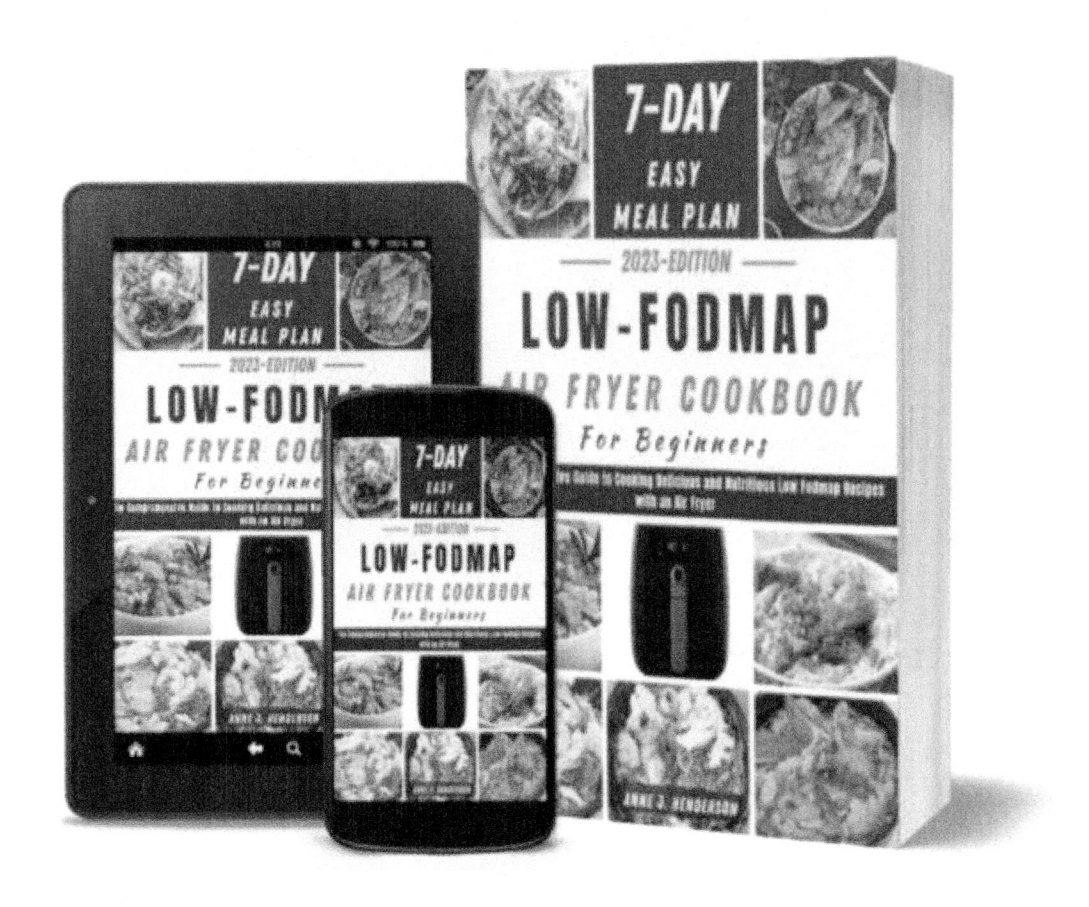

Table of content

INTRODUCTION 6
   Who is this book for? 7
   How can this book help you? 7
   How This Book Wants to Help People 8

Chapter 1 10
   Understanding Low FODMAP Diet 10

Chapter 2 14
   Understanding an Air Fryer 14
   How Does the Air Fryer Work 14
   The Benefits of Using an Air Fryer 15
   Tips for Cooking Low FODMAP Foods with an Air Fryer 16

Chapter 3 18
   7 Days Low Fodmap Meal plan 18
   Day 1 18
   Breakfast 18
   Lunch 18
   Dinner 18
   Day 2 19
   Breakfast 19
   Lunch 19
   Dinner 19
   Day 3 19
   Breakfast 19
   Lunch 19
   Dinner 19
   Day 4 19

Breakfast 19
Lunch 20
Dinner 20
Day 5 20
Breakfast 20
Lunch 20
Dinner 20
Day 6 20
Breakfast 20
Lunch 20
Dinner 20
Day 7 21
Breakfast 21
Lunch 21
Dinner 21

Chapter 4 22
Low Fodmap Air Fryer Breakfast Recipes 22
1. Low FODMAP Smoothie Bowls 22
2. Low FODMAP Donuts 24
3. Low FODMAP Muffins 25
4. Low FODMAP Granola Bars 27
5. Low FODMAP Fruit Salad 29
6. Low FODMAP Waffles 30
7. Low FODMAP Breakfast Sausage Patties 32
8. Low FODMAP Banana Bread 33
9. Low FODMAP Yogurt Parfaits 35
10. Low FODMAP Oatmeal 37
11. Low FODMAP French Toast Sticks 38
12. Low FODMAP Bagels 40
13. Low FODMAP Breakfast Burritos 42

14. Low FODMAP Blueberry Pancakes..43

15. Low FODMAP Hash Browns...45

Chapter 5..48

Low Fodmap Air Fryer Lunch Recipes..48

1. Low FODMAP Zucchini..48

2. Low FODMAP Carrots..49

3. Low FODMAP Veggie Nuggets..51

4. Low FODMAP Tilapia...52

5. Low FODMAP Turkey Burgers...54

6. Low FODMAP Salmon with Roasted Vegetables.....................55

7. Low FODMAP Quinoa Salad...57

8. Low FODMAP Lentil Soup..59

9. Low FODMAP Tofu..61

10. Low FODMAP Salmon..62

11. Low FODMAP Veggie Kabobs..64

12. Low FODMAP Chicken Wings...66

13. Low FODMAP Tortilla Pizzas..67

14. Low FODMAP Fish Sticks..69

15. Low FODMAP Chicken Tenders..71

Chapter 6..74

Low Fodmap Air Fryer Dinner Recipes.......................................74

1. Low FODMAP Halloumi...74

2. Low FODMAP Asparagus...75

3. Low FODMAP Sweet Potato Fries...77

4. Low FODMAP Roasted Vegetables.......................................78

5. Low FODMAP Brussels Sprouts...80

6. Low FODMAP Sweet Potato Fries...81

7. Low FODMAP Salmon with Lemon and Herbs.......................83

8. Low FODMAP Shrimp Scampi...84

9. Low FODMAP Chicken Breasts..86

10. Low FODMAP Pork Chops...88
11. Low FODMAP Turkey Burgers..89
12. Low FODMAP Sweet Potato Fries...91

Chapter 7..94
Low Fodmap Air Fryer Desserts Recipes..94
1. Low FODMAP Blueberry Muffins..94
2. Low FODMAP Lemon Bars...95
3. Low FODMAP Chocolate Mousse...97
4. Low FODMAP Chocolate Chip Cookies......................................98
5. Low FODMAP Popsicles..100
6. Low FODMAP Fruit Salad..101
7. Low FODMAP Yogurt Parfait...103
8. Low FODMAP Apples..104
9. Low FODMAP Peaches..106

Chapter 8..108
Low Fodmap Air Fryer Snacks Recipes...108
1. Low FODMAP Guacamole and veggies......................................108
2. Low FODMAP Pizza Dough..109
3. Low FODMAP Quesadillas..111
4. Low FODMAP Taquitos...112
5. Low FODMAP Pita Chips..114
6. Low FODMAP Popcorn...115
7. Low FODMAP Celery with Peanut Butter..................................117
8. Low FODMAP Apples with Peanut Butter..................................119
9. Low FODMAP Trail Mix..120

Conclusion..122

INTRODUCTION

Sara has been suffering with IBS for years. She had tried everything to relieve her symptoms, but nothing seemed to work. She was always bloated, constipated, or diarrhea, and she was starting to get really discouraged.

One day, Sara was chatting to her buddy about her IBS. Her buddy informed her about a low-FODMAP cookbook that she had been using. FODMAP stands for fermentable oligosaccharides, disaccharides, monosaccharides, and polyols.

These are short-chain carbohydrates that are poorly absorbed in the small intestine. In people with IBS, these carbohydrates can ferment in the large intestine, which can lead to symptoms like bloating, gas, diarrhea, and constipation.

Sara decided to give the low-FODMAP diet a try. She got the booklet and began following the recipes. At first, it was hard to change her eating habits. She missed her favorite meals, and she felt like she was constantly on a diet. But after a few weeks, she began to perceive a change. Her symptoms started to improve, and she felt more energetic.

Sara continued to follow the low-FODMAP diet for six months. During that period, her IBS symptoms subsided totally. She was able to consume a range of things without any issues. She was also able to shed weight and enhance her general health.

Sara is so grateful that she found the low-FODMAP diet. She says that it has changed her life. She is no longer embarrassed by her IBS symptoms, and she is able to live a normal life. She is also able to enjoy her favorite foods again, without any problems.

If you are suffering from IBS, I encourage you to try this low-FODMAP diet. It may just be the answer to your prayers.

Welcome To This Book "Low FODMAP Air Fryer Cookbook For Beginners"

If you're looking for a way to eat delicious, healthy food without suffering from the symptoms of IBS, then this book is for you. The Low Fodmap Air Fryer Cookbook for Beginners is filled with easy-to-follow recipes that are both low in FODMAPs and air-fried to perfection.

Who is this book for?

This book is for everyone especially beginners who wishes to enjoy tasty, nutritious cuisine without suffering from the symptoms of IBS. It is also a great resource for people who are new to the Low Fodmap Diet or who are looking for new ways to cook air-fried food.

How can this book help you?

This book can help you in a number of ways. It can assist you:

- Learn about the Low Fodmap Diet
- Find delicious, easy-to-make recipes that are low in FODMAPs

- Learn how to cook air-fried food
- Improve your overall health and well-being

How This Book Wants to Help People

This book was written with the intention of helping people who are struggling with IBS and other digestive disorders. We believe that everyone deserves to enjoy delicious, healthy food, and we hope that this book will help you to do just that.

We are committed to providing you with the best possible information and recipes, and we are always looking for ways to improve our book. If you have any feedback or suggestions, please feel free to contact us.

We hope that you will like this book!

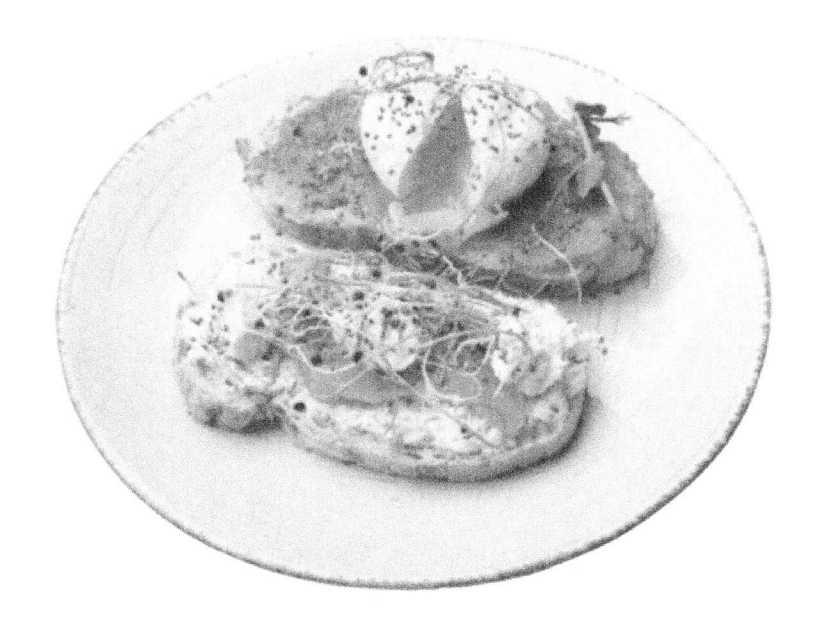

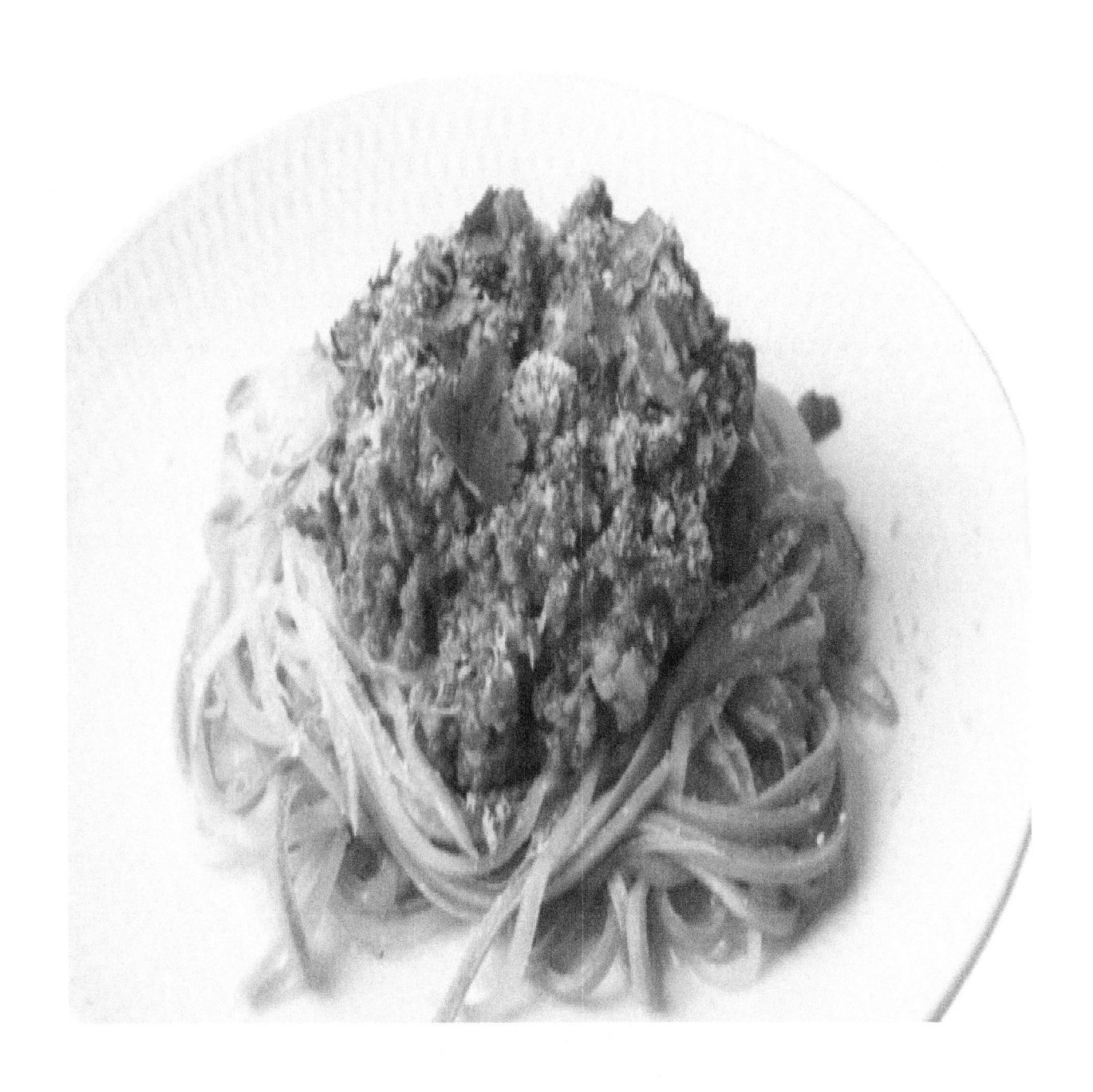

Low FODMAP Diet

Chapter 1

Understanding Low FODMAP Diet

A low FODMAP diet is a diet that restricts certain types of carbohydrates called fermentable oligosaccharides, disaccharides, monosaccharides, and polyols (FODMAPs). These carbohydrates are poorly absorbed in the small intestine, and they may induce symptoms such as bloating, gas, diarrhea, and constipation in persons with irritable bowel syndrome (IBS) and other functional gastrointestinal disorders.

The low FODMAP diet is a three-step process:

1. Elimination phase: This is the harshest phase of the diet, and it entails removing all high FODMAP items from your diet. This period normally lasts for two to six weeks.

2. Challenge phase: Once you have been on the elimination phase for two to six weeks, you may start to reintroduce high FODMAP foods one at a time to test whether they trigger your symptoms. This period normally lasts for two to six weeks.

3. Reintroduction phase: During this phase, you will continue to consume the low FODMAP foods that you tolerated during the challenge phase, and you will avoid the high FODMAP foods that you discovered to be troublesome. This phase is lifelong, and it allows you to customize your diet to fit your individual needs.

There are several resources available to help you follow a low FODMAP diet. The Monash University Low FODMAP Diet app is a great resource for finding low FODMAP foods and recipes. There are also numerous publications and websites that give information about the low FODMAP diet.

If you are considering following a low FODMAP diet, it is important to talk to your doctor or a registered dietitian. They can help you determine if the diet is right for you and can provide guidance on how to follow it safely.

Here are some of the advantages of adopting a low FODMAP diet:

1. Reduces symptoms of IBS: The low FODMAP diet has been demonstrated to be useful in lowering symptoms of IBS, such as bloating, gas, diarrhea, and constipation.

2. Improves quality of life: People who follow a low FODMAP diet often report an improvement in their quality of life, including less pain, less time spent in the bathroom, and more energy.

3. Is safe and effective: The low FODMAP diet is safe and effective for most individuals. However, it is vital to consult your doctor before beginning the regimen, particularly if you have any underlying health concerns.

If you are suffering symptoms of IBS or another functional gastrointestinal condition, speak to your doctor about if a low FODMAP diet may be good for you.

There are several advantages to adopting the low FODMAP diet. For people with IBS, the diet can significantly improve symptoms and improve quality of life. The diet can also help people with other digestive disorders, such as small intestinal bacterial overgrowth (SIBO), fructose malabsorption, and lactose intolerance.

In addition to improving digestive health, the low FODMAP diet can also have other benefits, such as:

1. Weight loss: The low FODMAP diet is naturally low in calories and fat, which may help individuals lose weight or maintain a healthy weight.

2. Improved gut health: The low FODMAP diet may assist to enhance the balance of bacteria in the gut, which can have a favorable influence on general health.

3. Reduced inflammation: The low FODMAP diet can help to reduce inflammation in the gut, which can benefit people with conditions such as IBS, Crohn's disease, and ulcerative colitis.

If you are considering following the low FODMAP diet, it is important to talk to your doctor or a registered dietitian. They can assist you to build a strategy that is ideal for you and can give support and direction throughout the process.

Here are some recommendations for following the low FODMAP diet:

- **Read food labels carefully:** Many foods contain hidden FODMAPs, thus it is crucial to check food labels carefully.

- **Cook at home:** When you cook at home, you can manage the ingredients and make sure that your meal is low in FODMAPs.

- **Be patient:** The low FODMAP diet can be challenging at first, but it is important to be patient and persistent. With time and effort, you can find a way to manage your symptoms and improve your quality of life.

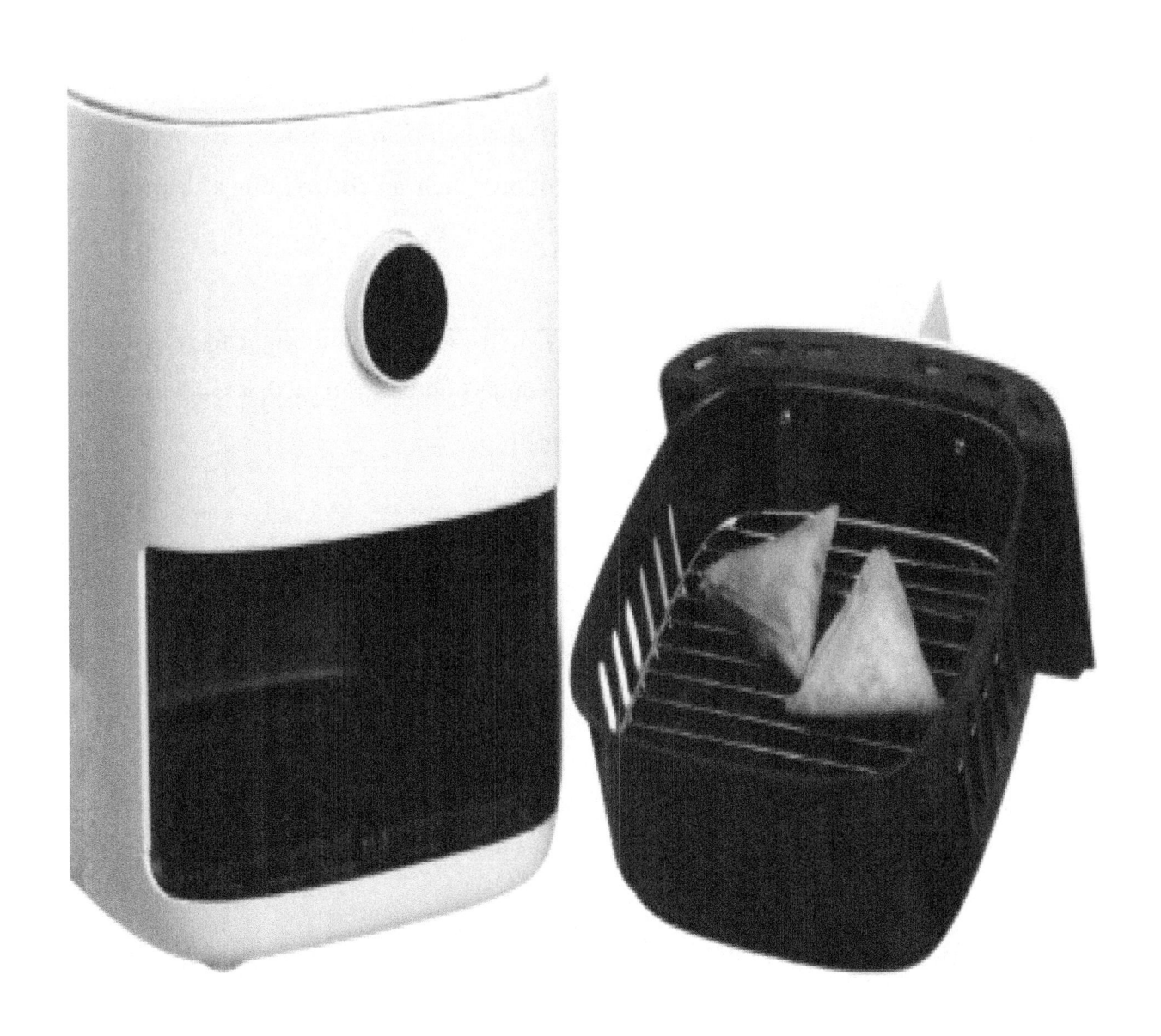

AIR FRYER

Chapter 2

Understanding an Air Fryer

An air fryer is a small kitchen appliance that cooks food by circulating hot air around it. Air fryers are a great way to cook healthy food because they don't require oil. This makes them a good option for people who are looking to reduce their fat intake or who have food allergies or sensitivities.

How Does the Air Fryer Work

Air fryers work by using a heating element to heat up the air inside the appliance. The hot air is then circulated around the food by a fan. This procedure generates a convection current, which cooks the food equally on all sides.

Air fryers can be used to cook a variety of foods, including french fries, chicken nuggets, fish sticks, vegetables, and even pizza. They are a great way to cook healthy meals without using a lot of oil.

Here are some of the benefits of using an air fryer:

- Cooks food fast and evenly
- Uses less oil than typical frying techniques
- Creates crispy, golden-brown food
- Can be used to cook a variety of foods
- Easy to clean

If you are looking for a healthy and convenient way to cook food, an air fryer is a great option.

Here are some suggestions for utilizing an air fryer:

- Preheat the air fryer according to the manufacturer's instructions.
- Don't overcrowd the air fryer. Food requires space to cook evenly.
- Shake the basket halfway through cooking to ensure that the food cooks evenly.
- Use a little layer of oil to prevent food from sticking.
- Check the food frequently to make sure that it is not overcooked.
- Air fryers can be a great way to cook healthy meals without using a lot of oil. However, it is important to use them safely and correctly.

Here are some safety tips to keep in mind:

- Always follow the manufacturer's instructions.
- Do not leave the air fryer alone while it is cooking.
- Do not use metal utensils in the air fryer.
- Do not overfill the air fryer.
- Be cautious while handling hot food.

With a little care and attention, air fryers may be a safe and convenient method to prepare meals.

The Benefits of Using an Air Fryer

Air fryers are a common kitchen gadget that cooks food using hot air circulation. They are often touted as a healthier alternative to deep frying, as they use less oil. Here are some of the perks of utilizing an air fryer:

1. Healthier cooking: Air fryers use less oil than deep fryers, which can help you reduce your intake of unhealthy fats. This can be a good option for people who are trying to lose weight or improve their heart health.

2. Quicker cooking: Air fryers may cook food quicker than regular ovens. This may be a time-saver, particularly if you are short on time.

3. Crispy food: Air fryers can create crispy, golden-brown food that is similar to deep-fried food. This is because the heated air travels over the food, generating a crispy surface without the need for a lot of oil.

4. Versatile: Air fryers can be used to cook a variety of foods, including chicken, fish, vegetables, and even frozen foods. This makes them a flexible kitchen device that can be used for a range of dishes.

5. Easy to use: Air fryers are generally easy to use and clean. Simply put your food in the basket, set the timer, and let the air fryer handle the rest.

Overall, air fryers are a handy and healthy method to prepare meals. If you are searching for a solution to lower your consumption of bad fats and cook meals quicker, an air fryer may be a suitable alternative for you.

Tips for Cooking Low FODMAP Foods with an Air Fryer

Here are some recommendations for cooking low FODMAP meals in an air fryer:

1. Choose the proper components. Not all foods are created equal when it comes to the low FODMAP diet. Some foods, such as garlic and onion, are high in FODMAPs, which can cause digestive problems in people with irritable bowel syndrome (IBS) and other conditions. When picking ingredients for your air fryer recipes, be sure to use low FODMAP-friendly ones.

2. Preheat your air fryer. Preheating your air fryer helps to guarantee that your food cooks evenly. Most air fryers need to be preheated to 350 degrees Fahrenheit.

3. Don't overcrowd the air fryer basket. Overcrowding the air fryer basket will prevent the food from cooking evenly. Be sure to leave enough space between each piece of food so that the air can circulate freely.

4. Shake or stir the food halfway through cooking. Shaking or shaking the food midway through cooking helps to ensure that it cooks evenly on all sides.

5. Cook the food until it is golden brown and crispy. The cooking time will vary depending on the type of food you are cooking. For example, chicken breasts may need to cook for 15-20 minutes, but french fries may just need to cook for 10-12 minutes.

6. Let the food cool slightly before serving. This will assist to avoid the meal from being overly hot and creating any intestinal pain.

With a little forethought, you can quickly make tasty and enjoyable low FODMAP meals with your air fryer.

Chapter 3

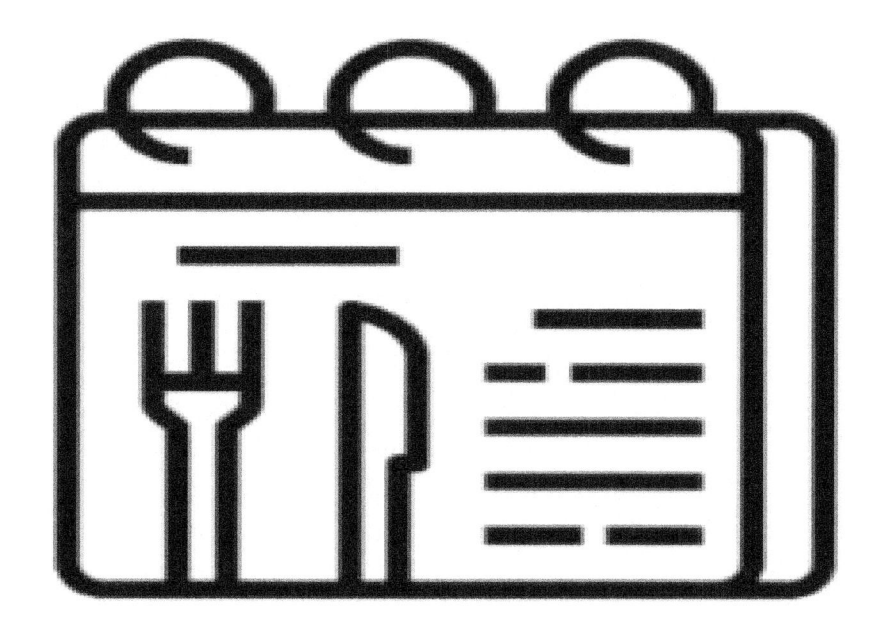

7 Days Low Fodmap Meal plan

Day 1

Breakfast

Air-fried tofu scramble with vegetables

Lunch

Air-fried salmon with roasted vegetables

Dinner

Air-fried chicken breast with quinoa and vegetables

Day 2

Breakfast

Air-fried oatmeal with berries

Lunch

Air-fried veggie burgers on whole-wheat buns

Dinner

Air-fried fish tacos with corn tortillas, cabbage, and salsa

Day 3

Breakfast

Air-fried frittata with cheese and vegetables

Lunch

Air-fried chickpeas with a side salad

Dinner

Air-fried chicken wings with your favorite dipping sauce

Day 4

Breakfast

Air-fried sweet potato hash with eggs

Lunch

Air-fried veggie nuggets with a side of hummus

Dinner

Air-fried steak with roasted vegetables

Day 5

Breakfast

Air-fried pancakes with fruit

Lunch

Air-fried veggie wraps with your favorite fillings

Dinner

Air-fried shrimp with rice and vegetables

Day 6

Breakfast

Air-fried French toast with maple syrup

Lunch

Air-fried chicken nuggets with a side of vegetables

Dinner

Air-fried fish with roasted potatoes

Day 7

Breakfast

Air-fried waffles with fruit

Lunch

Air-fried veggie burgers on whole-wheat buns

Dinner

Air-fried chicken breast with quinoa and vegetables

These are just a few ideas for low FODMAP recipes that can be made in an air fryer. With a little creativity, you can easily come up with your own delicious and healthy meals.

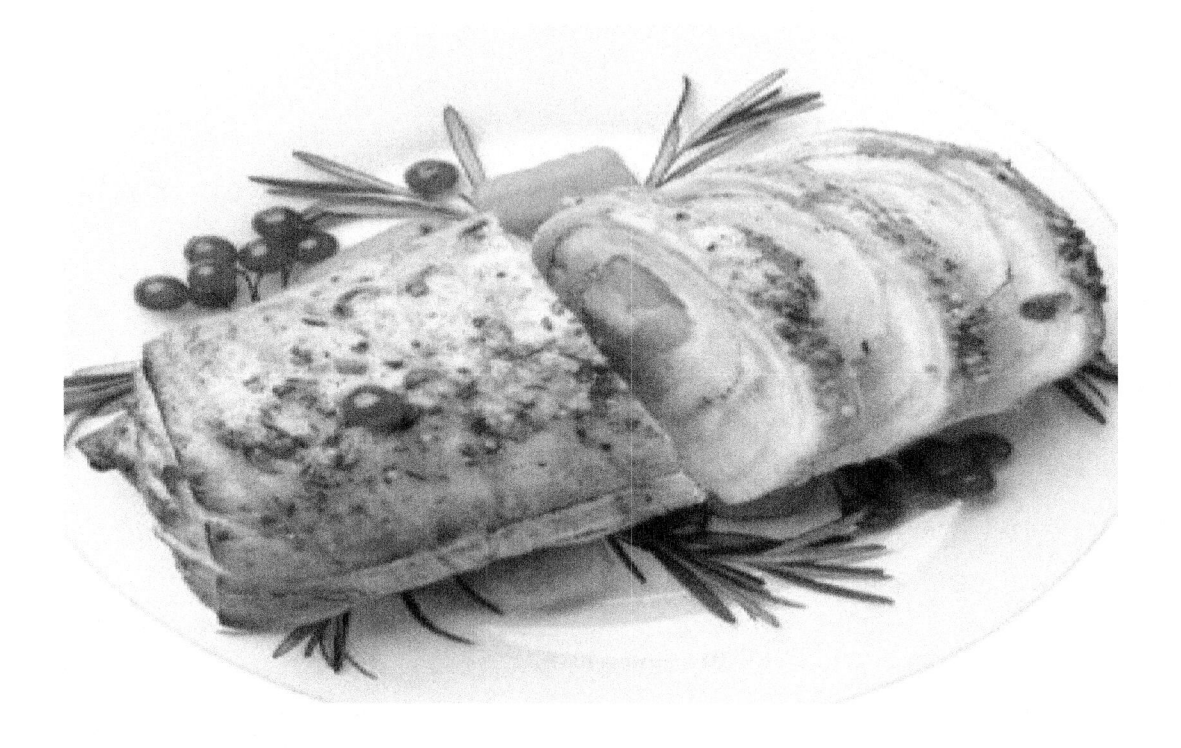

Chapter 4

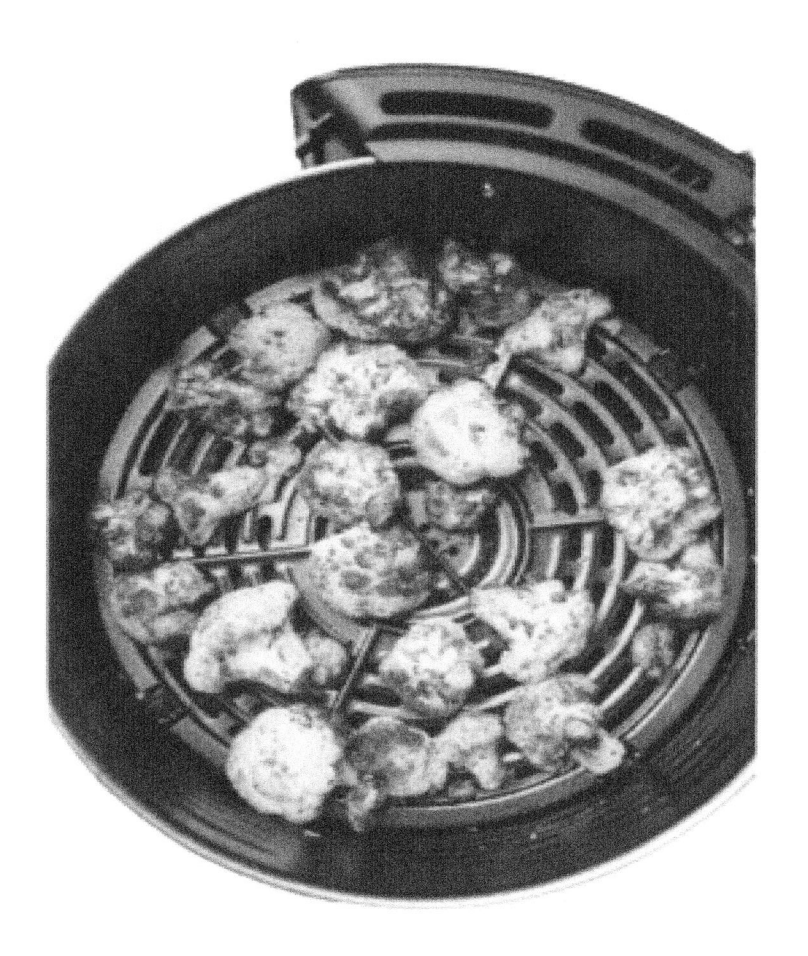

Low Fodmap Air Fryer Breakfast Recipes

1. Low FODMAP Smoothie Bowls

This recipe is for a delicious and nutritious smoothie bowl that is perfect for breakfast, lunch, or a snack. It is made with low FODMAP ingredients and cooked in an air fryer for a healthy and convenient option.

Preparation Time: 3 minutes
Cooking Time: 5-7 minutes, or until golden brown.
Total Time: 8-10 minutes

Ingredients:

- 1 cup low FODMAP milk
- 1/2 cup frozen berries
- 1/2 banana
- 1 scoop protein powder
- 1 tbsp chia seeds
- 1 tablespoon ground flaxseed
- 1/2 teaspoon vanilla extract
- Toppings: granola, fruit, nuts, seeds

Instructions:

- In a blender, mix all ingredients except for the toppings.
- Blend until smooth.
- Pour into a bowl and top with your preferred toppings.

Nutrition:

Here is a breakdown of the nutrition information for one serving of this recipe:

- Calories: 350
- Carbohydrates: 40 grams
- Fat: 10 grams
- Protein: 15 grams
- Fiber: 10 grams

Tips

- Feel free to use any type of low FODMAP milk in this recipe.

- You can also use other fruits in place of the berries.
- To make this dish vegan, use a plant-based milk and a vegan protein powder.
- For a gluten-free option, use gluten-free granola.

2. Low FODMAP Donuts

These low FODMAP doughnuts are a tasty and simple way to enjoy a sweet treat without having to worry about triggering your symptoms. They are manufactured with gluten-free flour, so they are also an excellent alternative for persons with celiac disease or gluten sensitivity.

Preparation time: 15 minutes
Cooking time: 10-12 minutes
Total time: 25-30 minutes

Ingredients:

- 1 cup gluten-free flour
- 1/2 cup sugar
- 1/2 teaspoon baking powder
- 1/2 teaspoon baking soda
- 1/4 teaspoon salt 2 big eggs
- 1/2 cup milk of choice
- 1/4 cup melted butter
- 1 teaspoon vanilla extract

Instructions:

- Preheat your air fryer to 350 degrees Fahrenheit.
- In a large bowl, whisk together the flour, sugar, baking powder, baking soda, and salt.
- In a separate bowl, whisk together the eggs, milk, butter, and vanilla extract.
- Add the wet ingredients to the dry ingredients and mix until just combined.

- Drop the dough by spoonfuls into the air fryer basket.
- Air fried for 10-12 minutes, or until golden brown.
- Let cool slightly before glazing or frosting.

Nutrition:

- Calories: 150
- Carbohydrates: 25 grams
- Fat: 6 grams
- Protein: 4 grams
- Fiber: 2 grams

Tips

- For a more flavorful donut, you can add 1/2 cup of chocolate chips or dried fruit to the batter.
- You may also prepare these donuts in a conventional oven. Preheat your oven to 350 degrees Fahrenheit and bake for 12-15 minutes, or until golden brown.
- To glaze the donuts, just whisk up 1 cup of powdered sugar, 1/4 cup of milk, and 1 teaspoon of vanilla essence. Dip the doughnuts in the glaze and allow them cool fully before serving.

3. Low FODMAP Muffins

These low FODMAP muffins are a delightful and simple way to enjoy a morning treat. They are created with gluten-free flour, almond milk, and blueberries, and they are fried in an air fryer for a quick and simple way to have a nutritious breakfast on the table.

Preparation time: 10 minutes
Cooking time: 15-20 minutes
Total time: 25-30 minutes

Ingredients:

- 1 cup gluten-free flour
- 1/2 cup almond milk
- 1/4 cup coconut oil, melted
- 1 egg
- 1 teaspoon baking powder
- 1/2 teaspoon baking soda
- 1/4 teaspoon salt
- 1/2 cup blueberries

Instructions:

- Preheat the air fryer to 350 degrees F.
- In a large bowl, mix together the flour, almond milk, coconut oil, egg, baking powder, baking soda, and salt.
- Fold in the blueberries.
- Divide the batter evenly among 12 muffin cups lined with paper liners.
- Air fried for 15-20 minutes, or until the muffins are golden brown and a toothpick inserted into the middle comes out clean.
- Let cool in the pan for a few minutes before removing to a wire rack to cool completely.

Nutrition Information:

- Calories: 150
- Carbohydrates: 20 grams
- Fat: 10 grams
- Protein: 5 grams
- Fiber: 3 grams

Tips

- For a sweeter muffin, add 1/4 cup of sugar to the batter.
- For a more tart muffin, add 1/2 cup of raspberries or blackberries to the batter.
- To make these muffins ahead of time, prepare the batter as directed and then chill it in the refrigerator for up to 24 hours. When you are ready to bake, preheat the air fryer and then bake the muffins according to the instructions.

These muffins can be stored in an airtight container at room temperature for up to 3 days.

4. Low FODMAP Granola Bars

Low FODMAP granola bars are a great way to get a healthy snack or breakfast on the go. They are also gluten-free and vegan, making them a fantastic alternative for anyone with dietary limitations. This dish is simple to follow and only takes around 30 minutes to create.

Preparation time: 10 minutes
Cooking time: 15-20 minutes
Total time: 25-30 minutes

Ingredients:

- 1 2/3 cups old-fashioned oats
- 1/2 cup dried cranberries
- 1/2 cup raisins
- 1/2 cup toasted pecans or walnuts, chopped
- 1/3 cup almond flour
- 1/4 cup unsweetened shredded coconut
- 1/4 cup sunflower seeds
- 1/2 teaspoon cinnamon
- 1/2 teaspoon salt
- 1/3 cup creamy, smooth peanut butter

- 1/3 cup sugar
- 1/3 cup vegetable oil, such as canola or safflower
- 1/4 cup maple syrup
- 2 teaspoons rice malt syrup
- 1 tablespoon water
- 1 teaspoon vanilla extract

Instructions:

- Preheat the air fryer to 350 degrees F (175 degrees C).
- In a large bowl, mix the oats, cranberries, raisins, pecans, almond flour, coconut, sunflower seeds, cinnamon, and salt.
- In a small bowl, whisk together the peanut butter, sugar, oil, maple syrup, rice malt syrup, and vanilla extract.
- Pour the wet ingredients into the dry ingredients and mix until well combined.
- Press the mixture into an 8x8 inch baking dish that has been lined with parchment paper.
- Bake in the air fryer for 15-20 minutes, or until the top is golden brown.
- Let cool completely before cutting into bars.

Nutrition:

One bar of these low FODMAP granola bars includes approximately:

- Calories: 190
- Carbohydrates: 26 grams
- Fat: 10 grams
- Protein: 4 grams
- Fiber: 4 grams

Tips

- For a chewier granola bar, bake for a longer length of time, or until the top is extremely dark brown.
- For a crunchier granola bar, bake for a shorter length of time.
- Feel free to add additional ingredients to the granola bar mixture, such as chocolate chips, almonds, or seeds.

These granola bars can be stored in an airtight container at room temperature for up to 1 week.

5. Low FODMAP Fruit Salad

This Low FODMAP Fruit Salad is a delicious and healthy way to enjoy a variety of fruits. The air fryer helps to caramelize the natural sugars in the fruit, giving it a delicious flavor and a slightly crispy texture. This salad is perfect for a light snack or dessert.

Preparation time: 10 minutes
Cooking time: 10-15 minutes
Total time: 20-25 minutes

Ingredients:

- 1 papaya, peeled and diced
- 1 pineapple, peeled, cored, and sliced
- 1 cantaloupe, peeled and diced 2 cups red grapes, halved

Instructions:

- Preheat the air fryer to 350 degrees Fahrenheit.
- In a large bowl, mix the papaya, pineapple, cantaloupe, and grapes.
- Air fried the fruit for 10-15 minutes, or until it is somewhat softened and caramelized.
- Serve immediately.

Nutrition Facts:

- Calories: 200
- Carbohydrates: 30 grams
- Fat: 0 grams
- Protein: 5 grams
- Fiber: 10 grams

Tips

- You can also use other low FODMAP fruits in this recipe, such as berries, peaches, or plums.
- If you don't have an air fryer, you may roast the fruit in the oven at 350 degrees Fahrenheit for 15-20 minutes.

6. Low FODMAP Waffles

These Low FODMAP Waffles are a delicious and easy-to-make breakfast option that is perfect for people with IBS or other digestive conditions. They are made with gluten-free flour, almond milk, and eggs, and they are cooked in an air fryer for a crispy and golden brown finish.

Preparation Time: 10 minutes
Cooking Time: 5 minutes each waffle creating 15 minutes for 3 waffle
Total Time: 25 minutes.

Ingredients:

- 1 cup gluten-free flour
- 1/2 cup almond milk
- 1 egg
- 1 tablespoon baking powder

- 1/4 teaspoon salt
- 1 tablespoon maple syrup
- 1/2 teaspoon vanilla extract

Instructions:

- In a large bowl, whisk together the flour, almond milk, egg, baking powder, and salt.
- Stir in the maple syrup and vanilla essence.
- Preheat the air fryer to 350 degrees Fahrenheit.
- Spray the air fryer basket with cooking spray.
- Pour 1/4 cup of batter onto the air fryer basket for each waffle.
- Cook the waffles for 5 minutes each side, or until golden brown.
- Repeat steps 5 and 6 until all of the batter is utilized.
- Serve the waffles warm with your preferred toppings.

Nutrition Information:

One waffle contains approximately:

- Calories: 150
- Carbohydrates: 25 grams
- Fat: 5 grams
- Protein: 5 grams
- Fiber: 2 grams

Tips

- For a sweeter waffle, add one additional tablespoon of maple syrup.
- For a more savory waffle, add 1/2 teaspoon of garlic powder and 1/4 teaspoon of onion powder to the batter.
- You can also use any type of milk you like in this recipe.

- If you don't have an air fryer, you can cook these waffles in a waffle iron. Just adjust the cooking time accordingly.

7. Low FODMAP Breakfast Sausage Patties

These low FODMAP breakfast sausage patties are a quick and simple way to start your day. They are made with ground pork, brown sugar, sage, thyme, salt, fennel seeds, chili powder, and paprika. The patties are fried in an air fryer, which gives them a crispy outside and a juicy inside.

Preparation Time: 5 minutes
Cooking Time: 10 minutes
Total Time: 15 minutes

Ingredients:

- 1 tablespoon firmly packed light brown sugar
- 1 tablespoon coarsely chopped fresh sage or 1 teaspoon rubbed (ground) sage
- 1 tablespoon coarsely chopped fresh thyme or 1 teaspoon dried thyme
- 1 1/4 tablespoons kosher salt
- 1 teaspoon crushed fennel seeds
- 1/2 teaspoon chili powder, such as ground red serrano chile
- 1/4 teaspoon paprika
- Freshly ground black pepper
- 1 pound (455 g) ground pork

Instructions:

- In a larger bowl, mix the brown sugar, sage, thyme, salt, fennel seeds, chili powder, paprika, and black pepper.

- Add the ground pork and stir until thoroughly blended.
- Form the mixture into eight 3-tablespoon sized balls.
- Flatten each ball into a 1/4-inch thick patty.
- Preheat the air fryer to 375 degrees Fahrenheit.
- Place the patties in the air fryer basket, allowing space between them.
- Air fry for 10 minutes, flipping halfway through, or until the patties are cooked through.
- Serve immediately.

Nutrition:

One serving (2 patties) of these low FODMAP breakfast sausage patties contains approximately:

- Calories: 200
- Carbohydrates: 10 grams
- Fat: 15 grams
- Protein: 15 grams
- Fiber: 1 gram

Tips

- If you don't have an air fryer, you may cook these patties in a pan over medium heat. Cook for 5-7 minutes each side, or until cooked through.
- You may also add additional ingredients to the sausage combination, such as chopped onion, garlic, or bell pepper.
- Serve these patties with your favorite breakfast dishes, such as eggs, pancakes, or waffles.

8. Low FODMAP Banana Bread

This recipe is for a delicious and moist banana bread that is also low in FODMAPs. It is manufactured with gluten-free flour, so it is also an excellent alternative for persons with celiac disease or gluten sensitivity. The banana bread is baked in an air fryer, which gives it a crunchy top and a soft, fluffy inside.

Preparation Time: 10 minutes
Cooking Time: 50-60 minutes
Total Time: 60-70 minutes

Ingredients:

- 1 1/2 cups (218 g) low FODMAP, gluten-free all-purpose flour
- 1 teaspoon baking soda
- 1/2 teaspoon salt
- 1/3 cup (75 ml) vegetable oil, such as canola
- 1/4 cup (50 g) sugar
- 1/4 cup (54 g) tightly packed light brown sugar
- 2 large eggs, at room temperature
- 1 1/2 cups (300 g) fork-mashed ripe banana (approximately 3 medium)
- 1 teaspoon vanilla extract
- 1 cup (99 g) toasted walnut or pecan halves, finely chopped (optional)

Instructions:

- Preheat the air fryer to 350 degrees Fahrenheit.
- Grease and flour a 7x5 inch loaf pan.
- In a large basin, mix together the flour, baking soda, and salt.
- In a separate bowl, whisk together the oil, sugar, brown sugar, eggs, and vanilla extract.
- Add the wet ingredients to the dry ingredients and stir until just mixed.
- Fold in the walnuts or pecans, if desired.
- Pour the batter into the prepared loaf pan and bake for 50-60 minutes, or until a toothpick inserted into the center comes out clean.

- Let the banana bread cool in the pan for 10 minutes before removing to a wire rack to cool completely.

Nutrition Information:

Per Serving (1/8 loaf)

- Calories: 180
- Carbohydrates: 25 grams
- Fat: 10 grams
- Protein: 4 grams
- Fiber: 2 grams

Tips

- For a deeper taste, use mashed ripe bananas that are little overripe.
- If you don't have an air fryer, you may bake the banana bread in a preheated oven at 350 degrees Fahrenheit for 50-60 minutes, or until a toothpick inserted into the middle comes out clean.
- The banana bread may be kept in an airtight jar at room temperature for up to 3 days. It may also be frozen for up to 2 months.

9. Low FODMAP Yogurt Parfaits

Low FODMAP yogurt parfaits are a delightful and easy-to-make breakfast or snack. They are created using gluten-free oats, yogurt, fruit, and honey. The air fryer helps to produce a crispy coating on the oats, while the yogurt and berries offer a creamy and refreshing touch.

Preparation Time: 10 minutes
Cooking Time: 5 minutes
Total Time: 15 minutes.

Ingredients:

- 1 cup gluten-free oats
- 1/2 cup yogurt
- 1/2 cup fruit, such as berries, peaches, or mango
- 1 tablespoon honey

Instructions:

- In a small dish, mix the oats and honey.
- Spread the oat mixture in the bottom of an air fryer basket.
- Cook in the air fryer at 350 degrees Fahrenheit for 5 minutes, or until the oats are golden brown and crispy.
- Top the oats with yogurt and fruit.
- Serve immediately.

Nutrition:

One serving of this dish comprises approximately:

- Calories: 250
- Carbohydrates: 35 grams
- Fat: 10 grams
- Protein: 10 grams
- Fiber: 5 grams

Tips

- For a more savory parfait, you may add spices such as cinnamon or nutmeg to the oat mixture.

- You can also use different types of fruit in this recipe. Some additional nice possibilities are blueberries, raspberries, and blackberries.
- If you don't have an air fryer, you may bake the oats in a preheated oven at 350 degrees Fahrenheit for 10 minutes, or until they are golden brown and crispy.

10. Low FODMAP Oatmeal

This recipe is a tasty and simple method to prepare oatmeal that is both low FODMAP and gluten-free. The oats are cooked in the air fryer, which gives them a slightly crispy texture that is very satisfying. The oatmeal is then sprinkled with your preferred toppings, such as fruit, nuts, or seeds.

Preparation Time: 5 minutes
Cooking Time: 10 minutes
Total Time: 15 minutes

Ingredients:

- 1/2 cup rolled oats
- 1/2 cup milk (any type)
- 1/2 teaspoon ground cinnamon
- 1/4 teaspoon ground ginger
- 1/4 teaspoon salt
- Optional toppings: fruit, nuts, seeds, honey, maple syrup

Instructions:

- In a small bowl, combine the oats, milk, cinnamon, ginger, and salt.
- Pour the mixture into the air fryer basket.
- Air fry at 350 degrees Fahrenheit for 10 minutes, or until the oats are cooked through.
- Serve immediately with your favorite toppings.

Nutritions:

- Calories: 200
- Carbohydrates: 25 grams
- Fat: 5 grams
- Protein: 5 grams
- Fiber: 5 grams

Tips

- For a thicker oatmeal, add 1/4 cup of water or milk to the mixture.
- To make the oatmeal ahead of time, cook it according to the instructions and then let it cool completely. Store it in an airtight jar in the refrigerator for up to 3 days. When you're ready to eat, warm the oats in the microwave or in the air fryer.
- Get creative with your toppings! Some additional fantastic possibilities are fruit, nuts, seeds, honey, maple syrup, or chocolate chips.

11. Low FODMAP French Toast Sticks

Low FODMAP French Toast Sticks are a tasty and simple way to enjoy a popular breakfast meal without the risk of triggering your symptoms. Made with gluten-free bread and a few basic ingredients, these sticks are great for anyone with IBS or other digestive disorders.

Preparation Time: 5 minutes
Cooking Time: 3-10 minutes
Total Time: 8-15 minutes

Ingredients:

- 2 slices gluten-free bread

- 1 egg
- 1/2 cup coconut milk
- 1 tablespoon coconut sugar
- 1 tablespoon ghee, melted
- 1/2 teaspoon vanilla extract
- 1/4 teaspoon cinnamon
- Cooking spray

Instructions:

- Preheat the air fryer to 370 degrees F.
- Cut each piece of bread into 3 sticks lengthwise.
- In a bowl, mix together the egg, coconut milk, coconut sugar, ghee, vanilla essence, and cinnamon.
- Working one at a time, dip each piece of bread into the egg mixture to coat on both sides.
- Generously spray the air fryer basket or rack with cooking spray.
- Lay the coated sticks in a single layer in the basket without touching each other.
- Air fry for 5 minutes, then flip with a spatula, and cook for another 3-5 minutes until golden brown and crispy. Keep a tight eye so they don't burn.
- Serve warm, with powdered sugar and/or maple syrup.

Nutrition Information:

One serving of Low FODMAP French Toast Sticks provides the following nutritional information:

- Calories: 200
- Carbohydrates: 25 grams
- Fat: 10 grams
- Protein: 7 grams
- Fiber: 2 grams

Tips

- For a more decadent treat, top the French toast sticks with your favorite toppings, such as whipped cream, chocolate chips, or fruit.
- If you don't have an air fryer, you can cook the French toast sticks in a conventional oven. Preheat the oven to 375 degrees F and bake for 10-12 minutes, or until golden brown and crispy.
- These French toast sticks are also a terrific alternative for a fast and simple snack or dessert.

12. Low FODMAP Bagels

These low FODMAP bagels are created with only three ingredients: gluten-free flour, yogurt, and baking powder. They are simple to create and cook in about 15 minutes in an air fryer. These bagels are great for a healthy breakfast or snack.

Preparation Time: 10 minutes
Cooking Time: 15 minutes
Total Time: 25 minutes

Ingredients:

- 1 cup gluten-free flour
- 1 cup yogurt (any flavor)
- 1 1/2 tablespoons baking powder
- 1/2 teaspoon salt
- Topping of your choice (optional)

Instructions:

- Preheat the air fryer to 350 degrees F.
- In a large basin, mix together the flour, yogurt, baking powder, and salt.
- Divide the dough into 4 equal pieces. Roll each piece into a ball.
- Use a rolling pin to flatten each ball into a 6-inch circle.
- Use a knife or a bagel cutter to cut a hole in the center of each circle.
- Place the bagels in the air fryer basket.
- Air fried the bagels for 10-12 minutes, or until they are golden brown and cooked through.
- Let the bagels cool slightly before serving.
- Top with your favorite toppings, such as cream cheese, butter, or cinnamon sugar.

Nutrition:

One bagel contains the following nutritional information:

- Calories: 150
- Carbohydrates: 25 grams
- Fat: 4 grams
- Protein: 5 grams
- Fiber: 4 grams

Tips

- If you don't have an air fryer, you can bake the bagels in a preheated oven at 350 degrees F for 15-20 minutes, or until they are golden brown and cooked through.
- You can experiment with different toppings, such as avocado, hummus, or peanut butter.
- These bagels are also fantastic for sandwiches or wraps.

13. Low FODMAP Breakfast Burritos

These low FODMAP breakfast burritos are a quick and easy way to start your day. They are produced using basic components that are easy to locate, and they may be tailored to your desire. The air fryer cooks the burritos uniformly and without any oil, making them a healthier alternative than frying.

Preparation Time: 15 minutes
Cooking Time: 10 minutes
Total Time: 25 minutes

Ingredients:

- 12 oz low FODMAP breakfast sausage, casings removed
- 3 Yukon gold potatoes, cut into tiny cubes
- 2 cups strong cheddar cheese, shredded 12 big eggs
- 1/2 cup lactose-free milk, 2%
- 1/4 teaspoon salt
- 1/8 teaspoon freshly ground pepper
- 12 6-inch low FODMAP tortillas

Instructions:

- Preheat the air fryer to 350 degrees Fahrenheit.
- In a large pan, saute the sausage over medium heat until browned. Drain off any excess fat.
- Add the potatoes to the skillet and cook until softened, about 5 minutes.
- In a medium bowl, mix together the eggs, milk, salt, and pepper.
- Add the sausage mixture, potatoes, and cheese to the egg mixture and whisk until completely incorporated.
- Divide the egg mixture evenly among the tortillas and roll up.

- Place the burritos in the air fryer and cook for 10 minutes, or until heated through.
- Serve immediately.

Nutrition Information Per burrito:

- Calories: 350
- Carbohydrates: 25 grams
- Fat: 15 grams
- Protein: 15 grams
- Fiber: 5 grams

Tips

- The air fryer time may vary depending on your air fryer model.
- For a hotter tortilla, add a sprinkle of cayenne pepper to the egg mixture.
- To make ahead, assemble the burritos without cooking them. Wrap them tightly in plastic wrap and refrigerate overnight. In the morning, cook them in the air fryer according to the instructions.

14. Low FODMAP Blueberry Pancakes

These low FODMAP blueberry pancakes are a tasty and simple way to enjoy a morning favorite without having to worry about triggering your symptoms. Made with gluten-free flour, almond milk, and eggs, these pancakes are also a great option for those with celiac disease or other gluten intolerances.

Preparation Time: 10 minutes
Cooking Time: 10 minutes
Total Time: 20 minutes

Ingredients:

- 1 cup gluten-free flour
- 1/2 teaspoon baking powder
- 1/4 teaspoon baking soda
- 1/4 teaspoon salt
- 1 egg
- 1/2 cup almond milk
- 1 tablespoon melted butter
- 1/2 cup blueberries

Instructions:

- In a bowl, whisk together the flour, baking powder, baking soda, and salt.
- In a separate dish, mix together the egg, almond milk, and melted butter.
- Add the wet ingredients to the dry ingredients and whisk until just combined.
- Fold in the blueberries.
- Heat your air fryer to 350 degrees Fahrenheit.
- Grease a baking pan with cooking spray.
- Pour 1/4 cup of batter onto each pancake in the baking pan.
- Air fry for 10 minutes, or until golden brown.
- Serve immediately.

Nutrition:

- Calories: 200
- Carbohydrates: 30 grams
- Fat: 10 grams
- Protein: 6 grams
- Fiber: 3 grams

Tips

- For a sweeter pancake, add 1 tablespoon of sugar to the batter.
- For a more flavorful pancake, add 1 teaspoon of vanilla extract to the batter.
- If you don't have an air fryer, you may cook these pancakes in a skillet on the stovetop. Heat a skillet over medium heat and cook the pancakes for 2-3 minutes each side, or until golden brown.

15. Low FODMAP Hash Browns

Low FODMAP hash browns are a tasty and simple way to enjoy a popular breakfast item without any of the digestive pain that might come with eating standard hash browns. This recipe is made with just a few simple ingredients and can be cooked in an air fryer, making it a quick and healthy option for any meal.

Preparation Time: 10 minutes
Cooking Time: 15-20 minutes
Total Time: 25-30 minutes

Ingredients:

- 2 big russet potatoes, peeled and grated
- 1 tablespoon olive oil
- 1/2 teaspoon salt
- 1/4 teaspoon black pepper

Instructions:

- Preheat the air fryer to 400 degrees Fahrenheit.
- In a large bowl, add the grated potatoes, olive oil, salt, and pepper.
- Toss to coat the potatoes evenly.

- Spread the potatoes in a single layer in the air fryer basket.
- Air fry for 15-20 minutes, or until the potatoes are golden brown and crispy.
- Serve immediately.

Nutrition Facts:

One serving of this dish (approximately 1/2 cup) gives the following nutritional information:

- Calories: 150
- Carbohydrates: 25 grams
- Fat: 10 grams
- Protein: 3 grams
- Fiber: 3 grams

Tips

- For extra crispy hash browns, blot the grated potatoes dry with paper towels before tossing them to the air fryer.
- If you don't have an air fryer, you can alternatively cook these hash browns in a pan over medium heat. Just be careful to fry them in batches so that they don't crowd the pan.
- Serve these hash browns with your favorite breakfast toppings, such as eggs, bacon, sausage, or cheese.

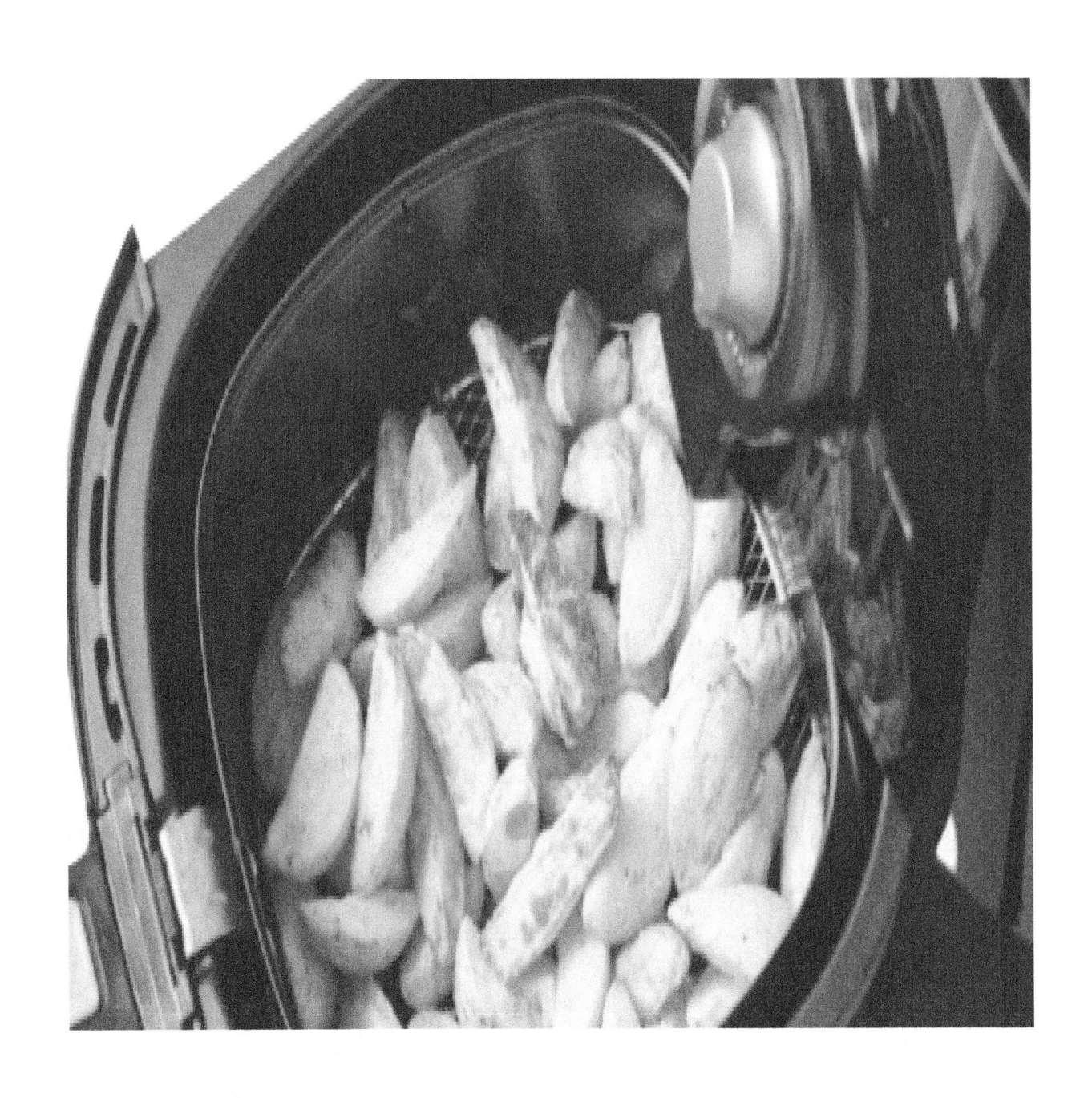

Low FODMAP Air Fryer Lunch Recipes

Chapter 5

Low Fodmap Air Fryer Lunch Recipes

1. Low FODMAP Zucchini

Zucchini is a low-calorie, high-fiber vegetable that is a great source of vitamins and minerals. It is also naturally gluten-free and low in FODMAPs, making it a good choice for people with digestive disorders. Air frying is a healthy cooking method that uses hot air to cook food, resulting in crispy, flavorful results with less oil.

Preparation Time: 5 minutes
Cooking Time: 10-12 minutes
Total Time: 15-17 minutes

Ingredients:

- 2 medium zucchini, sliced into
- 1/2-inch thick rounds
- 1 tablespoon olive oil
- 1/2 teaspoon salt
- 1/4 teaspoon black pepper

Instructions:

- Preheat the air fryer to 400 degrees F (200 degrees C).
- In a large bowl, stir together the zucchini, olive oil, salt, and pepper.
- Spread the zucchini in a single layer in the air fryer basket.
- Air fried for 10-12 minutes, or until the zucchini is soft and golden brown.
- Serve immediately.

Nutrition:

- Calories: 100
- Carbohydrates: 15 grams
- Fat: 5 grams
- Protein: 3 grams
- Fiber: 4 grams

Tips

- For extra crispy zucchini, sprinkle the zucchini with a spoonful of cornstarch before air fried.
- Serve the zucchini with your favorite dipping sauce, such as hummus, tzatziki, or ranch dressing.
- Air fried the zucchini in batches if required to avoid overcrowding.
- The cooking time may vary based on the size and thickness of your zucchini slices.

2. Low FODMAP Carrots

Air fryers are a terrific method to cook veggies without using a lot of oil. This recipe for Low FODMAP Carrots in an Air Fryer is a healthy and quick way to enjoy this delightful veggie.

Preparation Time: 5 minutes
Cooking Time: 15-20 minutes
Total Time: 20-25 minutes

Ingredients:

- 1 pound carrots, peeled and cut into 1-inch pieces
- 1 tablespoon olive oil
- 1/2 teaspoon salt
- 1/4 teaspoon black pepper

Instructions:

- Preheat the air fryer to 400 degrees Fahrenheit.
- In a large bowl, whisk together the carrots, olive oil, salt, and pepper.
- Spread the carrots in a single layer in the air fryer basket.
- Air fry for 15-20 minutes, or until the carrots are tender and slightly browned.
- Serve immediately.

Nutrition Information:

- Calories: 130
- Carbohydrates: 25 grams
- Fat: 6 grams
- Protein: 3 grams
- Fiber: 5 grams

Tips

- For a sweeter taste, add a spoonful of honey or maple syrup to the carrots before air frying.
- To add a little of fire, sprinkle the carrots with a dash of cayenne pepper before air frying.
- Serve the carrots with your favorite dipping sauce, such as ranch dressing or hummus.

Variations:

- Try using additional veggies in this dish, such as broccoli, Brussels sprouts, or sweet potatoes.
- For a more delicious recipe, add herbs and spices to the carrots before air frying. Some ideas include garlic powder, onion powder, paprika, or cumin.
- To make a bigger quantity of carrots, just double or quadruple the recipe.

3. Low FODMAP Veggie Nuggets

These low FODMAP veggie nuggets are a delicious and healthy alternative to traditional chicken nuggets. They are made with a variety of vegetables, including carrots, zucchini, and broccoli, and are coated in a gluten-free and grain-free breadcrumb mixture. They are then air fried until they are crispy and golden brown.

Preparation Time: 15 minutes
Cooking Time: 10 minutes
Total Time: 25 minutes

Ingredients:

- 1 cup grated carrots
- 1 cup grated zucchini
- 1 cup chopped broccoli florets
- 1/2 cup gluten-free and grain-free breadcrumbs
- 1/4 cup parmesan cheese, grated
- 1 egg, beaten
- 1 tablespoon olive oil
- 1 teaspoon salt
- 1/2 teaspoon black pepper

Instructions:

- Preheat the air fryer to 400 degrees Fahrenheit.
- In a large bowl, mix the carrots, zucchini, broccoli, breadcrumbs, parmesan cheese, egg, olive oil, salt, and pepper. Mix thoroughly to mix.
- Form the mixture into tiny nuggets.
- Air fry the nuggets for 10 minutes, or until they are crispy and golden brown.
- Serve immediately.

Nutrition:

- Calories: 150 per serving
- Carbohydrates: 15 grams
- Fat: 8 grams
- Protein: 10 grams
- Fiber: 4 grams

Tips

- You may use whatever sort of veggies that you prefer in these vegetarian nuggets.
- If you don't have an air fryer, you can bake these nuggets in the oven at 400 degrees Fahrenheit for 15-20 minutes, or until they are crispy and golden brown.
- Serve these nuggets with your favorite dipping sauce.

4. Low FODMAP Tilapia

Tilapia is a low-fat, high-protein fish that is a strong source of omega-3 fatty acids. It is also a naturally low FODMAP food, making it a suitable option for anyone following a low FODMAP diet. This recipe for air-fried tilapia is a quick and easy way to cook this healthy fish.

Preparation Time: 10 minutes
Cooking Time: 10-12 minutes
Total Time: 20-22 minutes

Ingredients:

- 1 pound tilapia fillets, skinless and boneless
- 1 tablespoon olive oil
- 1 teaspoon garlic powder
- 1/2 teaspoon salt

- 1/4 teaspoon black pepper

Instructions:

- Preheat the air fryer to 375 degrees F (190 degrees C).
- In a small bowl, add the olive oil, garlic powder, salt, and pepper.
- Brush the tilapia fillets with the olive oil mixture.
- Place the tilapia fillets in the air fryer basket and cook for 10-12 minutes, or until the fish is cooked through and flakes easily with a fork.
- Serve immediately.

Nutrition Information:

One serving of this dish comprises approximately:

- Calories: 180
- Carbohydrates: 10 grams
- Fat: 10 grams
- Protein: 20 grams
- Fiber: 0 grams

Tips

- For a more flavorful dish, you can add other seasonings to the olive oil mixture, such as onion powder, paprika, or chili powder.
- You can also add vegetables to the air fryer basket with the tilapia fillets. This is a great way to add extra nutrients to your meal.
- If you don't have an air fryer, you can cook the tilapia fillets in the oven. Preheat the oven to 400 degrees F (200 degrees C) and bake the tilapia fillets for 12-15 minutes, or until cooked through.

5. Low FODMAP Turkey Burgers

These low FODMAP turkey burgers are a tasty and simple way to enjoy a traditional American dinner. They are cooked using lean ground turkey, which is a rich source of protein and low in fat. The burgers are seasoned with a variety of herbs and spices, which gives them a tasty and juicy texture. They are cooked in an air fryer, which results in a crispy exterior and a moist interior.

Preparation time: 10 minutes
Cooking time: 10-12 minutes
Total time: 20-22 minutes

Ingredients:

- 1 pound lean ground turkey
- 1/2 cup chopped onion
- 1/4 cup chopped green bell pepper
- 1 egg
- 1 tablespoon Worcestershire sauce
- 1 tablespoon Dijon mustard
- 1 teaspoon garlic powder
- 1/2 teaspoon salt
- 1/4 teaspoon black pepper
- 4 low FODMAP burger buns
- Your favorite toppings, such as lettuce, tomato, cheese, and ketchup

Instructions:

- Preheat the air fryer to 375 degrees Fahrenheit.
- In a large bowl, mix the ground turkey, onion, bell pepper, egg, Worcestershire sauce, Dijon mustard, garlic powder, salt, and pepper. Mix until well combined.

- Form the ingredients into four equal-sized patties.
- Place the patties in the air fryer basket and cook for 10-12 minutes, or until cooked through.
- Serve on buns with your favorite toppings.

Nutrition Information:

- Calories: 250
- Carbohydrates: 10 grams
- Fat: 15 grams
- Protein: 20 grams
- Fiber: 3 grams

Tips

- For extra flavor, you can add a tablespoon of chopped fresh herbs, such as parsley or thyme, to the burger mixture.
- If you don't have an air fryer, you may cook the burgers in a pan over medium heat. Cook for 5-7 minutes each side, or until cooked through.

6. Low FODMAP Salmon with Roasted Vegetables

This dish is a tasty and nutritious way to eat salmon and veggies. The salmon is cooked in the air fryer, which results in a crispy exterior and juicy meat. The veggies are cooked with the fish, and they become soft and aromatic. This recipe is excellent for a fast and simple evening supper.

Preparation time: 10 minutes
Cooking time: 15-20 minutes
Total time: 25-30 minutes

Ingredients:

- 2 salmon fillets, approximately 6 ounces each
- 1 tablespoon olive oil
- 1/2 teaspoon salt
- 1/4 teaspoon black pepper
- 1/2 cup chopped onion
- 1/2 cup chopped red bell pepper
- 1/2 cup chopped green bell pepper
- 1/2 cup sliced zucchini
- 1/4 cup chopped fresh parsley

Instructions:

- Preheat the air fryer to 400 degrees F.
- In a small bowl, add the olive oil, salt, and pepper. Rub the mixture all over the salmon fillets.
- Place the salmon fillets in the air fryer basket.
- Add the onion, bell peppers, zucchini, and parsley to the air fryer basket around the salmon fillets.
- Air fry for 15-20 minutes, or until the salmon is cooked through and the veggies are soft.
- Serve immediately.

Nutrition:

- Calories: 370
- Carbohydrates: 10 grams
- Fat: 20 grams
- Protein: 30 grams
- Fiber: 3 grams

Tips

- If you don't have an air fryer, you may cook the salmon and veggies in the oven. Preheat the oven to 400 degrees F. Roast the salmon and veggies for 20-25 minutes, or until the fish is cooked through and the vegetables are soft.
- You may use any sort of veggies that you prefer in this dish. Some additional wonderful alternatives are broccoli, carrots, and potatoes.
- Serve this recipe with a side of rice or quinoa for a full supper.

7. Low FODMAP Quinoa Salad

This is a tasty and healthful salad that is excellent for a light lunch or supper. It is cooked using quinoa, which is a high-fiber, whole grain that is low in FODMAPs. The quinoa is cooked in an air fryer, which gives it a crunchy, somewhat smokey taste. The salad is then mixed with a variety of veggies, including red bell pepper, cucumber, tomato, and onion. A simple dressing prepared with olive oil, lemon juice, and herbs is added to complete the salad.

Preparation time: 10 minutes
Cooking time: 5-15 minutes
Total time: 15-25 minutes

Ingredients:

- 1 cup quinoa
- 1 cup water
- 1/2 cup red bell pepper, chopped
- 1/2 cup cucumber, diced
- 1/2 cup tomato, diced
- 1/2 onion, diced
- 2 tablespoons olive oil
- 2 teaspoons lemon juice

- 1 tablespoon chopped fresh herbs, such as parsley, basil, or thyme
- Salt and pepper to taste

Instructions:

- Rinse the quinoa in a fine mesh sieve until the water flows clear.
- In a small saucepan, mix the quinoa and water. Bring to a boil, then decrease heat to low and simmer for 15 minutes, or until the quinoa is cooked through.
- While the quinoa is cooking, warm the air fryer to 350 degrees Fahrenheit.
- Add the red bell pepper, cucumber, tomato, and onion to the air fryer basket.
- Air fry for 5-7 minutes, or until the veggies are soft and slightly browned.
- In a large bowl, mix the cooked quinoa, veggies, olive oil, lemon juice, herbs, salt, and pepper.
- Toss to blend and serve.

Nutrition:

One serving of this salad contains approximately:

- Calories: 250
- Carbohydrates: 35 grams
- Fat: 10 grams
- Protein: 9 grams
- Fiber: 5 grams

Tips

- For a more delicious salad, you may toast the quinoa before cooking it. To achieve this, just put the quinoa in a single layer on a baking sheet and toast in a preheated oven at 350 degrees Fahrenheit for 5-7 minutes, or until golden brown.

- You may use whatever sort of veggies you want in this salad. Some additional wonderful alternatives are broccoli, carrots, and zucchini.
- If you don't have an air fryer, you may cook the veggies in a pan on the stovetop. To cook this, heat a pan over medium heat and add the veggies. Cook for 5-7 minutes, or until tender and slightly browned.
- This salad is a terrific dinner prep alternative. You may prepare it ahead of time and preserve it in the refrigerator for up to 3 days.

8. Low FODMAP Lentil Soup

This tasty and easy-to-make soup is a fantastic way to get your daily dosage of fiber and protein. It is also low in FODMAPs, making it a healthy alternative for patients with irritable bowel syndrome (IBS). The soup is created with lentils, quinoa, veggies, and spices. It is cooked in an air fryer, which gives it a light and fluffy texture.

Preparation time: 10 minutes
Cooking time: 25-30 minutes
Total time: 35-40 minutes

Ingredients:

- 1 tablespoon olive oil
- 1 tablespoon garlic-infused olive oil
- 1 cup quinoa, washed
- 1 teaspoon ground ginger
- 1 teaspoon ground cumin
- 1 teaspoon ground coriander
- ½ teaspoon ground turmeric
- ¼ teaspoon ground cinnamon
- 8 cups water or low-FODMAP vegetable stock

- 1 big zucchini, chopped 2-3 medium carrots, chopped 1 can lentils, drained and washed thoroughly
- Salt to taste
- 1 bay leaf
- Pinch cayenne pepper (optional)

Instructions:

- Preheat the air fryer to 350 degrees Fahrenheit.
- Heat the olive oil and garlic-infused olive oil in a large pan over medium heat.
- Add the quinoa and simmer for 2-3 minutes, or until gently browned.
- Add the ginger, cumin, coriander, turmeric, and cinnamon and simmer for 1 minute longer.
- Add the water or stock, zucchini, carrots, lentils, salt, and bay leaf to the pan.
- Bring to a boil, then decrease heat to low and simmer for 20-25 minutes, or until the veggies are soft.
- Remove the bay leaf and toss in the cayenne pepper (if using).
- Serve hot.

Nutrition Facts:

One serving of this soup includes approximately:

- Calories: 250
- Carbohydrates: 40 grams
- Fat: 10 grams
- Protein: 10 grams
- Fiber: 10 grams

Tips

- For a richer soup, mash some of the lentils with a fork before serving.
- You may add additional veggies to the soup, such as potatoes, tomatoes, or mushrooms.
- Serve the soup with a dollop of sour cream or yogurt, or with a side of crusty bread.

9. Low FODMAP Tofu

This recipe is for a tasty and easy-to-make low FODMAP tofu dish that can be cooked in an air fryer. Air frying is a terrific technique to prepare tofu since it results in a crispy, delicious tofu that is still wet on the inside. This dish is also gluten-free and vegan.

Preparation Time: 10 minutes
Cooking Time: 20 minutes
Total Time: 30 minutes

Ingredients

- 1 block extremely firm tofu, pressed and cubed
- 1 tablespoon tamari
- 1 teaspoon sesame oil
- 2 tablespoons nutritional yeast
- 2 teaspoons cornstarch
- 1/2 cup veggies, such as broccoli, carrots, or peppers, chopped into bite-sized pieces

Instructions:

- In a large bowl, mix the tofu, tamari, sesame oil, nutritional yeast, and cornstarch. Mix thoroughly to coat the tofu.
- Preheat the air fryer to 375 degrees F (190 degrees C).
- Spread the tofu in a single layer in the air fryer basket.

- Air fried for 15-20 minutes, or until the tofu is golden brown and crispy.
- While the tofu is air frying, sauté the veggies in a skillet over medium heat.
- Serve the tofu with the veggies and enjoy!

Nutrition:

One serving of this dish comprises approximately:

- Calories: 423
- Carbohydrates: 59 grams
- Fat: 13 grams
- Protein: 22 grams
- Fiber: 10 grams

Tips

- You may use whatever sort of tofu you desire for this dish. However, super firm tofu is excellent for obtaining a crispy texture.
- If you don't have an air fryer, you may bake the tofu in the oven at 400 degrees F (200 degrees C) for 20-25 minutes, or until golden brown and crispy.
- You may alter the quantity of veggies you use to your preference.
- You may also add additional ingredients to the tofu, such as garlic powder, onion powder, or chili powder.
- This meal is an excellent source of protein and fiber. It is also gluten-free and vegan.

10. Low FODMAP Salmon

Salmon is a tasty and healthful seafood that is low in FODMAPs, making it a wonderful alternative for those with irritable bowel syndrome (IBS). Air frying is a healthier technique to prepare salmon than standard frying, since it requires less oil. This dish is fast and simple to prepare, and it provides perfectly cooked salmon with a crispy exterior.

Preparation Time: 10 minutes

Cooking Time: 10-15 minutes

Total Time: 20-25 minutes

Ingredients:

- 4 salmon fillets, approximately 6 ounces each
- 1 tablespoon olive oil
- 1 teaspoon salt
- 1/2 teaspoon black pepper
- 1/4 teaspoon garlic powder
- 1/4 teaspoon paprika

Instructions:

- Preheat your air fryer to 375 degrees Fahrenheit.
- In a small bowl, add the olive oil, salt, pepper, garlic powder, and paprika.
- Brush the salmon fillets with the olive oil mixture.
- Place the salmon fillets in the air fryer basket and cook for 10-12 minutes, or until the fish is cooked through and flakes readily with a fork.
- Serve immediately.

Nutrition Information:

One serving of this dish comprises approximately:

- Calories: 250
- Carbohydrates: 1 gram
- Fat: 15 grams
- Protein: 20 grams
- Fiber: 0 grams

Tips

- If you don't have an air fryer, you may cook the salmon in a preheated oven at 400 degrees Fahrenheit for 12-15 minutes, or until the salmon is cooked through and flakes easily with a fork.
- You may also add additional herbs and spices to the olive oil combination, such as thyme, rosemary, or lemon zest.
- Serve the salmon with your favorite sides, such as roasted veggies, rice, or quinoa.

11. Low FODMAP Veggie Kabobs

This dish is a terrific way to get your daily intake of veggies in a fun and savory manner. The veggies are cooked in an air fryer, which gives them a crispy surface and a soft inside. The kabobs are also low in FODMAPs, making them a fantastic alternative for anyone with digestive difficulties.

Preparation Time: 15 minutes
Cooking Time: 20 minutes
Total Time: 35 minutes

Ingredients:

- 1 big zucchini, cut into 1-inch cubes
- 1 yellow squash, cut into 1-inch cubes
- 1 red bell pepper, cut into 1-inch chunks
- 1 green bell pepper, cut into 1-inch cubes
- 1 onion, sliced into 1-inch chunks
- 1 tablespoon olive oil
- 1 teaspoon salt
- 1/2 teaspoon black pepper

- 12 wooden skewers, soaking in water for 30 minutes

Instructions:

- Preheat the air fryer to 400 degrees Fahrenheit.
- In a large bowl, add the zucchini, yellow squash, bell peppers, onion, olive oil, salt, and pepper. Toss to coat.
- Thread the veggies onto the skewers, rotating between various kinds of vegetables.
- Place the skewers in the air fryer and cook for 15-20 minutes, or until the veggies are soft and slightly browned.
- Serve immediately.

Nutritional Information:

- Calories: 150
- Carbohydrates: 15 grams
- Fat: 10 grams
- Protein: 5 grams
- Fiber: 5 grams

Tips

- For a more delicious kebab, you may marinate the veggies in a combination of olive oil, lemon juice, garlic, and herbs for at least 30 minutes before cooking.
- You may also add additional veggies to the kebabs, such as mushrooms, tomatoes, or carrots.
- If you don't have wooden skewers, you may use metal skewers. Just make sure to cover them with cooking spray before adding the veggies to prevent them from sticking.

12. Low FODMAP Chicken Wings

These low FODMAP chicken wings are a tasty and simple way to enjoy a popular snack without any digestive problems. The air fryer process guarantees that the wings are crispy and juicy on the inside, while the low FODMAP seasoning gives them a tasty kick.

Preparation time: 10 minutes
Cooking time: 20-25 minutes
Total time: 30-35 minutes

Ingredients:

- 1 pound chicken wings, split at the joints
- 1 tablespoon olive oil
- 1 teaspoon garlic powder
- 1/2 teaspoon onion powder
- 1/2 teaspoon smoked paprika
- 1/4 teaspoon salt
- 1/4 teaspoon black pepper

Instructions:

- Preheat the air fryer to 400 degrees Fahrenheit.
- In a large bowl, add the chicken wings, olive oil, garlic powder, onion powder, smoked paprika, salt, and black pepper. Toss to coat evenly.
- Place the chicken wings in the air fryer basket in a single layer.
- Air fried for 20-25 minutes, or until the chicken is cooked through and the skin is crispy.
- Serve immediately with your favorite dipping sauce.

Nutrition:

One serving (approximately 6 wings) of these low FODMAP chicken wings includes the following nutritional information:

- Calories: 250
- Carbohydrates: 10 grams
- Fat: 15 grams
- Protein: 20 grams
- Fiber: 0 grams

Tips

- For extra crispy wings, sprinkle them with a little bit of cornstarch before air frying.
- To prepare a low FODMAP buffalo sauce, mix 1/2 cup hot sauce, 1/4 cup butter, and 1 tablespoon apple cider vinegar in a small skillet. Heat over medium heat until the butter is melted and the sauce is creamy.
- Serve the chicken wings with your favorite dipping sauce, such as blue cheese dressing, ranch dressing, or honey mustard sauce.

13. Low FODMAP Tortilla Pizzas

Low FODMAP Tortilla Pizzas are a fast and simple way to enjoy a tasty and fulfilling pizza without the risk of provoking any digestive issues. Made with basic ingredients and baked in an air fryer, these pizzas are ready in only a few minutes.

Preparation time: 10 minutes
Cooking time: 4-5 minutes
Total time: 14-15 minutes

Ingredients:

- 1 big corn tortilla
- 2 teaspoons low FODMAP pizza sauce
- 1/2 cup shredded mozzarella cheese
- Your favorite toppings, such as pepperoni, sausage, mushrooms, onions, peppers, etc.

Instructions:

- Preheat your air fryer to 400 degrees Fahrenheit.
- Spray the air fryer basket with non-stick cooking spray.
- Place the tortilla in the air fryer basket.
- Spread the pizza sauce over the tortilla.
- Top with the shredded mozzarella cheese and your preferred toppings.
- Air fried for 4-5 minutes, or until the cheese is melted and bubbling.
- Let cool for a few minutes before slicing and serving.

Nutrition Information:

One serving of Low FODMAP Tortilla Pizzas comprises approximately:

- Calories: 250
- Carbohydrates: 30 grams
- Fat: 10 grams
- Protein: 10 grams
- Fiber: 3 grams

Tips

- For a crispier crust, prepare a baking sheet in the oven at 400 degrees Fahrenheit. Place the tortilla on the prepared baking sheet before adding the pizza sauce and toppings. Air fried for a further 1-2 minutes, or until the crust is golden brown.
- If you don't have an air fryer, you may bake these pizzas in a preheated oven at 400 degrees Fahrenheit for 10-12 minutes, or until the cheese is melted and bubbling.
- Get creative with your toppings! There are countless alternatives when it comes to cooking Low FODMAP Tortilla Pizzas. Try using various varieties of cheese, veggies, and meats. You may also add a dab of olive oil or balsamic vinegar for a little of added flavor.

14. Low FODMAP Fish Sticks

These low FODMAP fish sticks are a tasty and nutritious alternative to regular fish sticks. They are produced using cod fillets that are covered in a crispy batter and then air fried to perfection. The outcome is a light and flaky fish stick that is excellent for a fast and simple weekday supper.

Preparation time: 15 minutes
Cooking time: 10-12 minutes
Total time: 25-30 minutes

Ingredients:

- 1 pound cod fillets, cut into 1-inch pieces
- 1/2 cup gluten-free all-purpose flour
- 1/2 teaspoon salt
- 1/4 teaspoon black pepper
- 1 egg, beaten
- 1 cup gluten-free panko bread crumbs
- 1/2 cup shredded low FODMAP potato chips

Instructions:

- Preheat the air fryer to 400 degrees Fahrenheit.
- In a shallow bowl, mix the flour, salt, and pepper.
- In a separate shallow dish, beat the egg.
- In a third shallow dish, mix the panko bread crumbs and crushed potato chips.
- Dip each piece of cod in the flour mixture, then the egg mixture, then the panko bread crumb mixture.
- Place the coated fish sticks in the air fryer basket in a single layer.
- Air fried for 10-12 minutes, or until golden brown and cooked through.
- Serve immediately with your favorite dipping sauce.

Nutrition:

One serving of these fish sticks comprises approximately:

- Calories: 200
- Carbohydrates: 15 grams
- Fat: 10 grams
- Protein: 20 grams
- Fiber: 2 grams

Tips

- For a more tasty fish stick, you may add herbs and spices to the flour mixture. Some excellent possibilities are garlic powder, onion powder, paprika, and cayenne pepper.
- If you don't have an air fryer, you may bake these fish sticks in the oven. Preheat the oven to 400 degrees Fahrenheit and bake for 15-20 minutes, or until golden brown and cooked through.

- Serve these fish sticks with your favorite dipping sauce, such as tartar sauce, ketchup, or ranch dressing.

15. Low FODMAP Chicken Tenders

Air fryers are a terrific method to cook chicken tenders without all the oil and fat of conventional frying. This recipe is for low FODMAP chicken tenders that are crispy and tasty.

Preparation Time: 10 minutes
Cooking Time: 10-12 minutes
Total Time: 20-22 minutes

Ingredients:

- 1 pound boneless, skinless chicken breasts, cut into 1-inch strips
- 1/2 cup gluten-free flour
- 1 teaspoon salt
- 1/2 teaspoon black pepper
- 1/2 cup gluten-free panko breadcrumbs
- 1 egg, beaten
- 1 tablespoon olive oil

Instructions:

- Preheat the air fryer to 375 degrees Fahrenheit.
- In a shallow bowl, mix the flour, salt, and pepper.
- In another shallow dish, mix the panko breadcrumbs.
- In a third shallow dish, mix together the egg and olive oil.
- Dip the chicken strips in the flour mixture, then the egg mixture, then the breadcrumb mixture.
- Place the chicken strips in the air fryer basket in a single layer.

- Cook for 10-12 minutes, or until the chicken is cooked through and the coating is golden brown.
- Serve immediately with your favorite dipping sauce.

Nutritional Information:

One serving of this dish (3 chicken tenders) includes approximately:

- Calories: 250
- Carbohydrates: 15 grams
- Fat: 10 grams
- Protein: 20 grams
- Fiber: 1 gram

Tips

- To make the chicken tenders even more crispy, you may spray them with a small amount of cooking spray before cooking.
- You may also add additional ingredients to the breadcrumb mixture, such as garlic powder, onion powder, or paprika.
- If you don't have an air fryer, you may cook the chicken tenders in the oven at 400 degrees Fahrenheit for 15-20 minutes, or until they are cooked through.

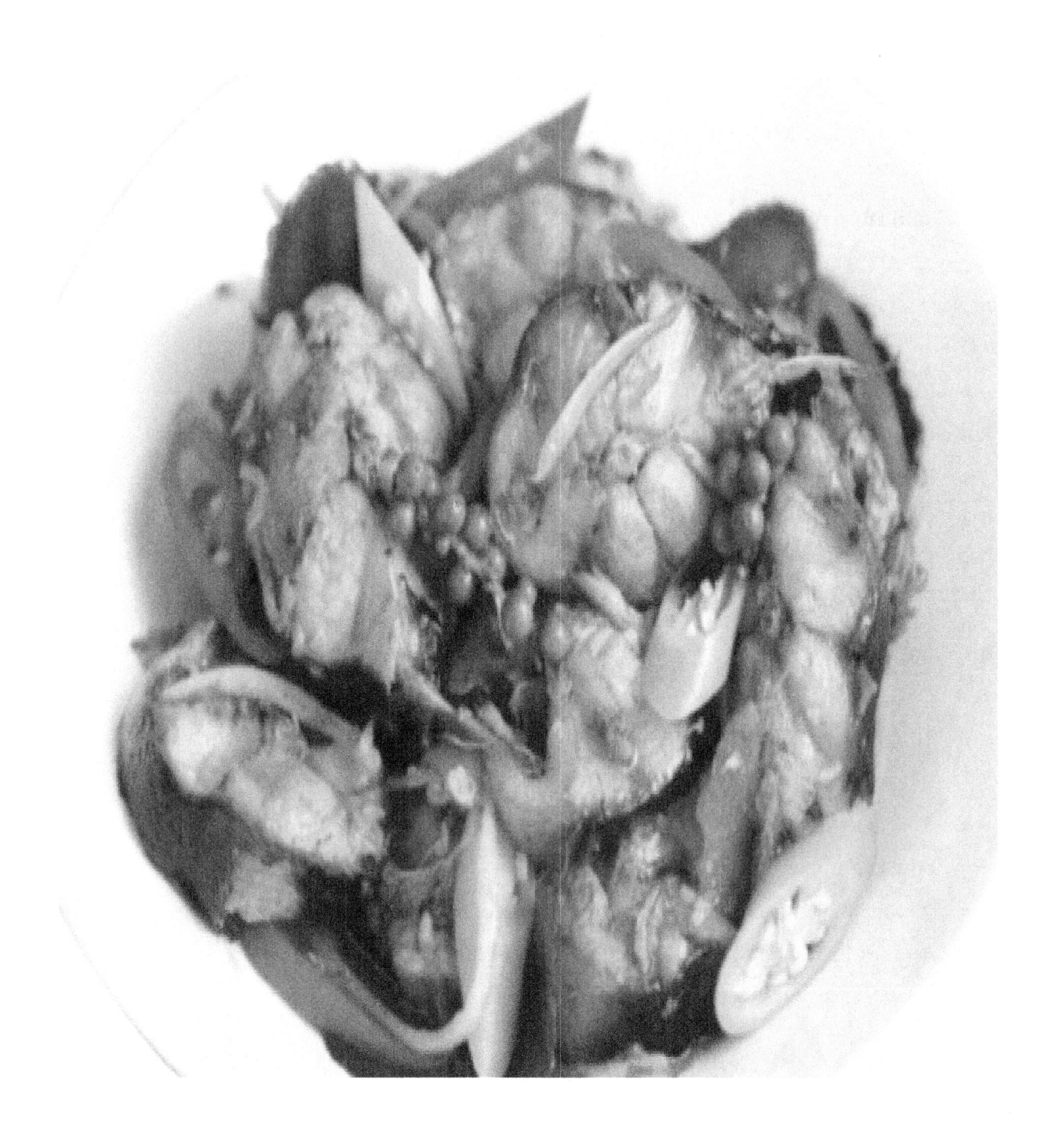

Low FODMAP Air Fryer Dinner Recipes

Chapter 6

Low Fodmap Air Fryer Dinner Recipes

1. Low FODMAP Halloumi

Halloumi is a kind of cheese that is naturally low in FODMAPs, making it a perfect alternative for persons with irritable bowel syndrome (IBS) or other digestive disorders. It is also an excellent source of protein and calcium.

Preparation Time: 5 minutes
Cooking Time: 10 minutes
Total Time: 15 minutes

Ingredients:

- 1 block of halloumi cheese, sliced into 1-inch chunks
- 1/4 cup all-purpose flour
- 1 egg, beaten
- 1/2 cup breadcrumbs
- 1 tablespoon olive oil

Instructions:

- Preheat the air fryer to 375 degrees F (190 degrees C).
- In a small bowl, mix the flour and 1/2 teaspoon salt.
- In a separate shallow dish, beat the egg.
- In a third shallow dish, mix the breadcrumbs and 1/2 teaspoon salt.
- Dip the halloumi cubes in the flour mixture, then the egg mixture, and finally the breadcrumb mixture.

- Drizzle the halloumi cubes with the olive oil.
- Air fried the halloumi cubes for 8-10 minutes, or until golden brown and crispy.
- Serve immediately with your favorite dipping sauce.

Nutrition Facts:

- Calories: 230
- Carbohydrates: 6 grams
- Fat: 15 grams
- Protein: 15 grams
- Fiber: 0 grams

Tips

- For a more savory crust, you may add your preferred herbs and spices to the breadcrumb mixture.
- You may also air fry halloumi skewers or bits. To achieve this, just thread the halloumi cubes onto skewers or toothpicks before coating and air frying.
- Air fried halloumi is an excellent snack or appetizer. It may also be served as a main meal with a side salad or veggies.

2. Low FODMAP Asparagus

Asparagus is a tasty and nutritious vegetable that is low in FODMAPs, making it a wonderful option for persons with irritable bowel syndrome (IBS). Air frying is a healthier technique to prepare asparagus, since it requires less oil than typical frying methods. This recipe is fast and simple to create, and the results are crispy, delicate asparagus that is excellent for a side dish or light entrée.

Preparation Time: 10 minutes
Cooking Time: 10-12 minutes

Total Time: 20-22 minutes

Ingredients:

- 1 pound fresh asparagus, trimmed
- 1 tablespoon olive oil
- 1/2 teaspoon salt
- 1/4 teaspoon black pepper

Instructions:

- Preheat your air fryer to 400 degrees Fahrenheit.
- In a large bowl, stir together the asparagus, olive oil, salt, and pepper.
- Spread the asparagus in a single layer in the air fryer basket.
- Air fry for 10-12 minutes, or until the asparagus is crisp and gently golden.
- Serve immediately.

Nutrition Information:

One serving of this dish (1/2 cup) includes the following nutritional information:

- Calories: 60
- Carbohydrates: 10 grams
- Fat: 4 grams
- Protein: 4 grams
- Fiber: 3 grams

Tips

- For a more delicious asparagus, you may add additional herbs and spices to the olive oil combination, such as garlic powder, onion powder, or Italian seasoning.

- If you don't have an air fryer, you may alternatively cook the asparagus in the oven. Preheat your oven to 400 degrees Fahrenheit and roast the asparagus for 15-20 minutes, or until tender and gently browned.
- Asparagus is a versatile vegetable that may be prepared in a number of ways. Try it as a side dish with grilled chicken or fish, or add it to a salad or stir-fry.

3. Low FODMAP Sweet Potato Fries

Air fryers are a terrific method to make healthy, crispy fries without all the oil. This recipe for Low FODMAP Sweet Potato Fries is simple to prepare and only takes around 30 minutes from start to finish.

Preparation Time: 10 minutes
Cooking Time: 15-20 minutes
Total Time: 25-30 minutes

Ingredients:

- 2 big sweet potatoes, peeled and cut into ¼-inch thick fries
- 1 tablespoon olive oil
- ½ teaspoon paprika
- ½ teaspoon garlic powder
- ½ teaspoon salt
- ¼ teaspoon black pepper

Instructions:

- Preheat your air fryer to 400 degrees Fahrenheit.
- In a large bowl, combine the sweet potato fries with the olive oil, paprika, garlic powder, salt, and pepper.
- Spread the fries in a single layer in the air fryer basket.

- Cook for 15-20 minutes, or until the fries are golden brown and crispy.
- Serve immediately and enjoy!

Nutrition Information:

- Calories: 180
- Carbohydrates: 30 grams
- Fat: 8 grams
- Protein: 3 grams
- Fiber: 4 grams

Tips

- For extra crispy fries, soak the sweet potato fries in cold water for 30 minutes before frying.
- If your air fryer is tiny, you may need to cook the fries in batches.
- Serve the fries with your preferred dipping sauce.

Variations

- For a sweeter taste, add 1 teaspoon of sugar to the dry ingredients.
- For a hotter taste, add ¼ teaspoon of cayenne pepper to the dry ingredients.
- For a more Mediterranean taste, add 1 teaspoon of dried oregano and 1 teaspoon of dried thyme to the dry ingredients.

4. Low FODMAP Roasted Vegetables

This dish is a terrific way to enjoy roasted veggies without the effort of heating up your oven. The air fryer cooks the veggies rapidly and evenly, so they come out wonderfully crispy and tasty. This dish is also low in FODMAPs, making it a wonderful alternative for patients with irritable bowel syndrome (IBS).

Preparation time: 10 minutes

Cooking time: 15-20 minutes

Total time: 25-30 minutes

Ingredients:

- 1 tablespoon olive oil
- 1 teaspoon garlic powder
- 1/2 teaspoon salt
- 1/4 teaspoon black pepper
- 1 pound vegetables, such as carrots, broccoli, Brussels sprouts, or cauliflower, chopped into bite-sized portions

Instructions:

- Preheat the air fryer to 400 degrees Fahrenheit.
- In a large bowl, add the olive oil, garlic powder, salt, and pepper.
- Add the veggies to the bowl and toss to coat.
- Spread the veggies in a single layer in the air fryer basket.
- Air fry for 15-20 minutes, or until the veggies are soft and slightly browned.
- Serve immediately.

Nutrition:

- Calories: 150
- Carbohydrates: 20 grams
- Fat: 10 grams
- Protein: 5 grams
- Fiber: 5 grams

Tips

- For a more delicious dinner, add your preferred herbs and spices to the veggies before air frying.
- If you are short on time, you may roast the veggies in the oven at 400 degrees Fahrenheit for 20-25 minutes.
- Serve the roasted veggies with your favorite protein and a side of rice or quinoa for a full dinner.

5. Low FODMAP Brussels Sprouts

Brussels sprouts are a wonderful and healthy vegetable that can be prepared in a number of ways. Air frying is a terrific technique to prepare Brussels sprouts because it creates crispy, delicious results without the need for extra oil. This recipe for Low FODMAP Brussels Sprouts in an Air Fryer is easy to prepare and only requires a few minutes of prep time.

Preparation time: 10 minutes
Cooking time: 15-20 minutes
Total time: 25-30 minutes

Ingredients:

- 1 pound Brussels sprouts, trimmed and halved
- 1 tablespoon olive oil
- 1/2 teaspoon salt
- 1/4 teaspoon black pepper

Instructions:

- Preheat the air fryer to 400 degrees F (200 degrees C).
- In a large bowl, stir together the Brussels sprouts, olive oil, salt, and pepper.

- Spread the Brussels sprouts in a single layer in the air fryer basket.
- Air fry for 15-20 minutes, or until the Brussels sprouts are soft and crispy.
- Serve immediately.

Nutrition Information:

One serving of this recipe (1/2 cup) includes approximately:

- Calories: 100
- Carbohydrates: 15 grams
- Fat: 5 grams
- Protein: 5 grams
- Fiber: 4 grams

Tips

- For a more savory meal, you may add extra ingredients to the Brussels sprouts, such as garlic powder, onion powder, or paprika.
- If you don't have an air fryer, you may roast the Brussels sprouts in the oven at 400 degrees F (200 degrees C) for 20-25 minutes, or until soft and crispy.
- Brussels sprouts are a fantastic source of fiber, which may assist to keep you feeling full and pleased. They are also a strong source of vitamins C and K.

6. Low FODMAP Sweet Potato Fries

Air fryer sweet potato fries are a delicious and healthy alternative to traditional fried french fries. They are produced with low FODMAP ingredients and are cooked in an air fryer, which results in crispy fries without all the oil.

Preparation Time: 10 minutes
Cooking Time: 15-20 minutes

Total Time: 25-30 minutes

Ingredients:

- 2 big sweet potatoes, peeled and cut into
- ¼-inch thick fries
- 2 tablespoons olive oil
- 1 teaspoon garlic powder
- 1 teaspoon onion powder
- 1 teaspoon salt
- ½ teaspoon black pepper

Instructions:

- Preheat your air fryer to 400 degrees Fahrenheit.
- In a large bowl, mix the sweet potato fries, olive oil, garlic powder, onion powder, salt, and pepper. Toss to coat evenly.
- Add the coated sweet potato fries to the air fryer basket and spread them out in a single layer.
- Air fry for 15-20 minutes, or until the fries are golden brown and crispy.
- Serve immediately and enjoy!

Nutrition Information:

- Calories: 160
- Carbohydrates: 25 grams
- Fat: 10 grams
- Protein: 4 grams
- Fiber: 4 grams

Tips

- For extra crispy fries, preheat your oven to 400 degrees Fahrenheit and bake the fries for an additional 5-10 minutes after air frying.
- If you don't have an air fryer, you can bake the sweet potato fries in a preheated oven at 400 degrees Fahrenheit for 20-25 minutes, or until golden brown and crispy.
- Serve with your favorite dipping sauce, such as ketchup, ranch dressing, or hummus.

7. Low FODMAP Salmon with Lemon and Herbs

Salmon is a delicious and healthy fish that is low in FODMAPs. This recipe is a simple and straightforward method to cook salmon in an air fryer. The lemon and herbs provide a touch of flavor and brightness, making this dish a terrific weekday supper.

Preparation Time: 10 minutes
Cooking Time: 15 minutes
Total Time: 25 minutes

Ingredients:

- 1 pound salmon fillet, skin on 1 tablespoon olive oil
- 1 lemon, zested and juiced
- 1 teaspoon dried thyme
- 1/2 teaspoon salt
- 1/4 teaspoon black pepper

Instructions:

- Preheat the air fryer to 400 degrees Fahrenheit.
- In a small bowl, combine the olive oil, lemon zest, lemon juice, thyme, salt, and pepper.
- Brush the salmon fillet with the olive oil mixture.

- Place the salmon fillet in the air fryer basket.
- Air fried for 15 minutes, or until the fish is cooked through.
- Serve immediately.

Nutrition:

- Calories: 270
- Carbohydrates: 1 gram
- Fat: 17 grams
- Protein: 25 grams
- Fiber: 0 grams

Tips

- If you don't have an air fryer, you may bake the salmon in a preheated oven at 400 degrees Fahrenheit for 15-20 minutes, or until cooked through.
- You may also add additional herbs and spices to the olive oil combination, such as rosemary, oregano, or garlic powder.
- Serve the salmon with your favorite sides, such as roasted veggies, rice, or quinoa.

8. Low FODMAP Shrimp Scampi

Shrimp scampi is a famous Italian dish that is often cooked with shrimp, garlic, butter, and white wine. This recipe for low FODMAP shrimp scampi is done in an air fryer, which makes it a healthier and quicker choice than conventional techniques.

Preparation Time: 10 minutes
Cooking Time: 5-7 minutes
Total Time: 15-17 minutes

Ingredients:

- 1 pound shrimp, peeled and deveined
- 1 tablespoon olive oil 2 cloves garlic, minced
- 1/2 cup dry white wine
- 1/4 cup chicken broth
- 1/4 cup chopped fresh parsley
- 1/4 teaspoon salt
- 1/4 teaspoon black pepper

Instructions:

- Preheat the air fryer to 400 degrees F (200 degrees C).
- In a large bowl, combine the shrimp with the olive oil, garlic, white wine, chicken broth, parsley, salt, and pepper.
- Place the shrimp in the air fryer basket in a single layer.
- Air fry for 5-7 minutes, or until the shrimp are pink and cooked through.
- Serve immediately with your favorite pasta or rice.

Nutrition Information:

One serving of this dish comprises approximately:

- Calories: 200
- Carbohydrates: 10 grams
- Fat: 10 grams
- Protein: 20 grams
- Fiber: 1 gram

Tips

- If you don't have an air fryer, you can also make this recipe in a skillet on the stovetop. Simply heat the olive oil in a large skillet over medium heat. Add the shrimp and heat for 2-3 minutes each side, or until pink and cooked through. Add the garlic, white wine, chicken broth, parsley, salt, and pepper and cook for 1-2 minutes more, or until the sauce has thickened. Serve immediately.
- You can also add other vegetables to this recipe, such as zucchini, mushrooms, or bell peppers.
- This dish is a fantastic source of protein and low in carbs, making it a healthy alternative for anyone with dietary restrictions.

9. Low FODMAP Chicken Breasts

Air fryers are a terrific method to cook chicken breasts fast and effortlessly. They utilize heated air to circulate over the meal, which results in crispy skin and juicy meat. This recipe is for low FODMAP chicken breasts that are seasoned with a basic combination of herbs and spices.

Preparation time: 5 minutes
Cooking time: 15-20 minutes
Total time: 20-25 minutes

Ingredients:

- 2 boneless, skinless chicken breasts
- 1 tablespoon olive oil
- 1 teaspoon salt
- 1/2 teaspoon black pepper
- 1 teaspoon smoked paprika
- 1 teaspoon dried oregano

Instructions:

- Preheat the air fryer to 360 degrees Fahrenheit.
- In a small bowl, mix the olive oil, salt, pepper, smoked paprika, and oregano.
- Brush the chicken breasts with the olive oil mixture.
- Place the chicken breasts in the air fryer basket and cook for 15-20 minutes, or until cooked through.
- Serve immediately.

Nutrition:

(Per serving)

- Calories: 250
- Carbohydrates: 2 grams
- Fat: 15 grams
- Protein: 30 grams
- Fiber: 0 grams

Tips

- For extra crispy chicken, cover the chicken breasts in a thin coating of breadcrumbs before air frying.
- To prevent the chicken breasts from adhering to the air fryer basket, spray the basket with a non-stick cooking spray.
- Serve the chicken breasts with your favorite sides, such as rice, veggies, or salad.

10. Low FODMAP Pork Chops

Air fryers are a great way to cook pork chops because they cook them evenly and quickly, without the need for added fat. This recipe is for low FODMAP pork chops, which implies that they are suitable for persons with irritable bowel syndrome (IBS) or other digestive issues.

Preparation time: 5 minutes
Cooking time: 10-12 minutes
Total time: 15-17 minutes

Ingredients:

- 4 boneless, pork chops, about 1 inch thick
- 1 tablespoon olive oil
- 1 teaspoon salt
- 1/2 teaspoon black pepper
- 1/2 teaspoon garlic powder
- 1/4 teaspoon paprika

Instructions:

- Preheat the air fryer to 375 degrees F (190 degrees C).
- In a small bowl, add the olive oil, salt, pepper, garlic powder, and paprika.
- Rub the spice mixture all over the pork chops.
- Place the pork chops in the air fryer basket and cook for 10-12 minutes, or until cooked through.
- Serve immediately.

Nutritional Information:

One serving of this meal (one pork chop) includes approximately:

- Calories: 240
- Carbohydrates: 0 grams
- Fat: 14 grams
- Protein: 24 grams
- Fiber: 0 grams

Tips

- For extra crispy pork chops, you can coat them in a mixture of breadcrumbs and parmesan cheese before cooking.
- If you don't have an air fryer, you can cook the pork chops in a preheated oven at 400 degrees F (200 degrees C) for 15-20 minutes, or until cooked through.
- Serve the pork chops with your favorite sides, such as roasted veggies, mashed potatoes, or rice.

11. Low FODMAP Turkey Burgers

These low FODMAP turkey burgers are a terrific way to have a tasty and nutritious lunch. They are cooked using lean ground turkey, which is a rich source of protein and low in fat. The burgers are also seasoned with low FODMAP components, such as scallions, Worcestershire sauce, and garlic-infused oil.

Preparation time: 10 minutes
Cooking time: 10-12 minutes
Total time: 20-22 minutes

Ingredients:

- 1 big egg

- 1 pound (455 g) 94% lean ground turkey 2 tablespoons sliced onions, green portions only 1 teaspoon Worcestershire sauce
- 1 tablespoon + 1 teaspoon low FODMAP garlic-infused oil, divided ½ teaspoon Bell's Seasoning
- Kosher salt
- Freshly ground black pepper
- 4 low FODMAP rolls
- Low FODMAP condiments of choice
- Sliced tomato and lettuce (optional)

Instructions:

- Preheat the air fryer to 375 degrees Fahrenheit.
- In a large bowl, mix the ground turkey, egg, scallions, Worcestershire sauce, 1 tablespoon of the garlic-infused oil, Bell's Seasoning, salt, and pepper. Mix thoroughly to mix.
- Form the ingredients into 4 equal-sized patties.
- Brush the patties with the remaining 1 teaspoon of garlic-infused oil.
- Air fried the patties for 10-12 minutes, or until cooked through.
- Serve on the low FODMAP buns with your preferred sauces and toppings.

Nutrition:

One burger includes approximately:

- Calories: 250
- Carbohydrates: 10 grams
- Fat: 15 grams
- Protein: 20 grams
- Fiber: 3 grams

Tips

- For a more savory burger, you may add extra spices, such as paprika, cumin, or chili powder.
- If you don't have an air fryer, you may cook the burgers in a pan or on the grill.
- Serve the burgers with your favorite toppings, such as ketchup, mustard, cheese, bacon, or avocado.

12. Low FODMAP Sweet Potato Fries

Sweet potato fries are a tasty and healthful alternative to standard french fries. They are abundant in fiber and vitamins, and they are also gluten-free and low in FODMAPs. This dish is simple to prepare and only takes around 30 minutes to cook.

Preparation time: 10 minutes
Cooking time: 15-20 minutes
Total time: 25-30 minutes

Ingredients:

- 1 big sweet potato, peeled and cut into fries
- 1 tablespoon olive oil
- 1/2 teaspoon salt
- 1/4 teaspoon black pepper
- 1/4 teaspoon garlic powder
- 1/4 teaspoon onion powder

Instructions:

- Preheat your air fryer to 400 degrees Fahrenheit.

- In a large bowl, stir together the sweet potato fries, olive oil, salt, pepper, garlic powder, and onion powder.
- Spread the sweet potato fries in a single layer in the air fryer basket.
- Air fry for 15-20 minutes, or until the sweet potato fries are golden brown and crispy.
- Serve immediately and enjoy!

Nutrition:

One serving of Low FODMAP Sweet Potato Fries in an Air Fryer includes the following nutrients:

- Calories: 150
- Carbohydrates: 25 grams
- Fat: 10 grams
- Protein: 4 grams
- Fiber: 5 grams

Tips

- For extra crispy fries, soak the sweet potato fries in cold water for 30 minutes before air frying.
- If your air fryer is tiny, you may need to cook the sweet potato fries in batches.
- Serve the sweet potato fries with your favorite dipping sauce, such as ketchup, ranch dressing, or blue cheese dressing.

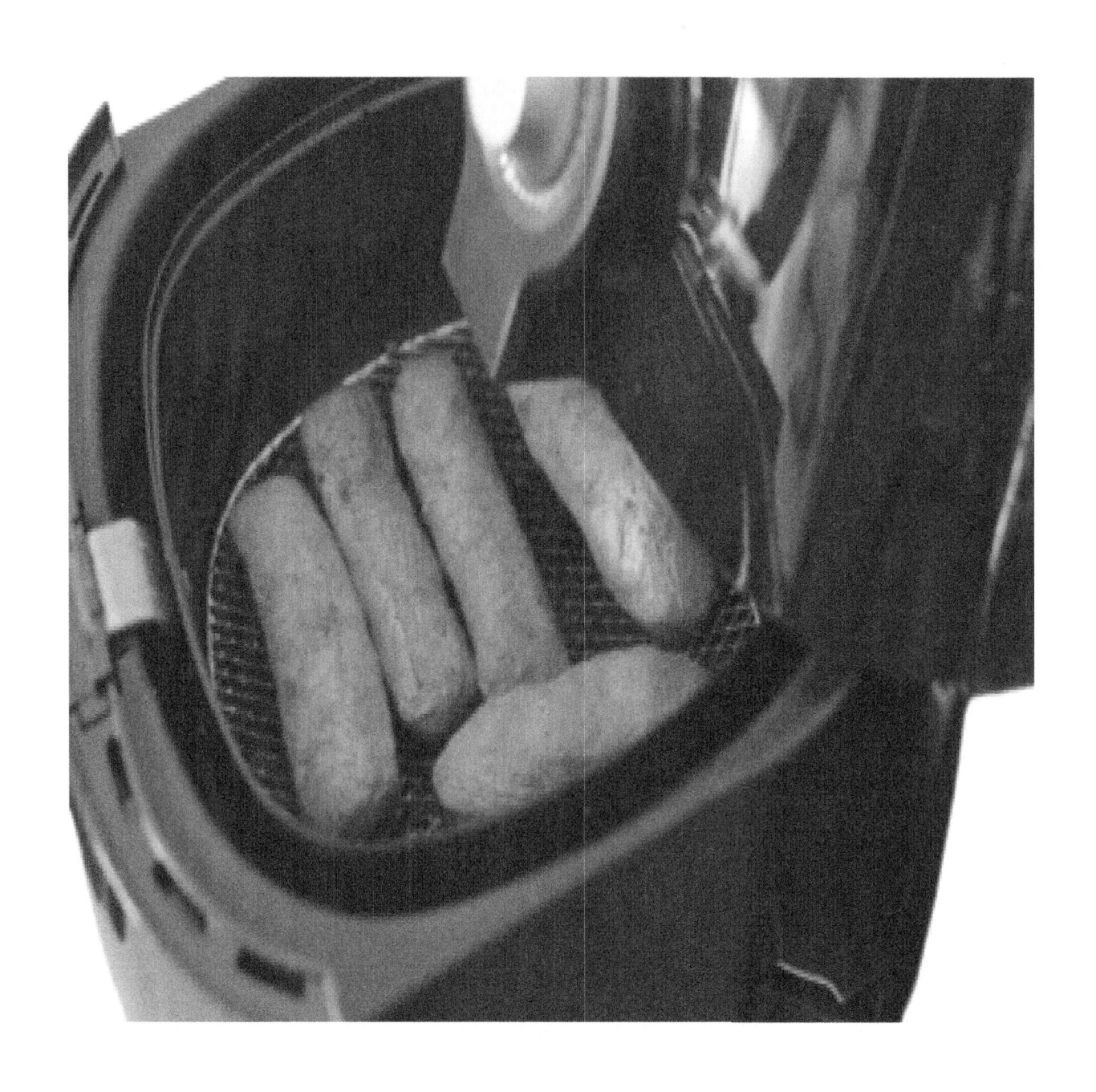

Low FODMAP Air Fryer Desserts Recipes

Chapter 7

Low Fodmap Air Fryer Desserts Recipes

1. Low FODMAP Blueberry Muffins

These low FODMAP blueberry muffins are a tasty and simple way to enjoy a sweet treat without feeling bloated or uncomfortable. They are manufactured with gluten-free flour, so they are also an excellent alternative for persons with celiac disease or gluten sensitivity.

Preparation time: 15 minutes
Cooking time: 12-15 minutes
Total time: 27-30 minutes

Ingredients:

- 2 cups low FODMAP gluten-free all-purpose flour
- 2 tablespoons baking powder
- 1/2 teaspoon salt
- 1/2 cup (1 stick; 113 g) unsalted butter, softened and cut into pieces
- 1 cup plus 2 teaspoons sugar, divided
- 2 teaspoons vanilla extract
- 2 big eggs, at room temperature
- 1/2 cup (120 ml) lactose-free whole milk, at room temperature
- 2 1/4 cups (383 g) fresh blueberries

Instructions:

- Preheat the air fryer to 350 degrees F (175 degrees C).
- In a large bowl, mix together the flour, baking powder, and salt.

- In a separate dish, beat together the butter and 1 cup of sugar until light and fluffy. Beat in the vanilla extract.
- Add the eggs one at a time, beating thoroughly after each addition.
- Add the flour mixture to the wet ingredients alternately with the milk, starting and finishing with the flour.
- Fold in the blueberries.
- Line a 6-cup muffin tray with paper liners.
- Fill each muffin liner approximately 2/3 full of batter.
- Bake in the air fryer for 12-15 minutes, or until a toothpick inserted into the middle of a muffin comes out clean.
- Let cool in the pan for a few minutes before transferring to a wire rack to cool fully.

Nutrition Information:

- Calories: 230
- Carbohydrates: 32 grams
- Fat: 11 grams
- Protein: 5 grams
- Fiber: 3 grams

2. Low FODMAP Lemon Bars

These low FODMAP lemon bars are a delightful and simple treat that is excellent for anybody following a low FODMAP diet. The acidic lemon filling is topped with a buttery shortbread crust, and the entire thing is fried in an air fryer for a fast and simple dessert.

Preparation Time: 15 minutes
Cooking Time: 25 minutes
Total Time: 40 minutes

Ingredients:

- 1 cup gluten-free flour
- ½ cup granulated sugar
- ½ cup unsalted butter, cold and cubed
- 4 big eggs
- ½ cup freshly squeezed lemon juice (approximately 3 lemons)
- ½ cup granulated sugar
- Powdered sugar, for sprinkling

Instructions:

- Preheat the air fryer to 325 degrees F.
- In a larger bowl, mix the flour and sugar. Cut in the butter until the mixture resembles coarse crumbs.
- Press the crumb mixture into the bottom of a 9x13 inch baking dish.
- In a large bowl, mix together the eggs, lemon juice, and sugar until thoroughly blended.
- Pour the lemon filling over the crust and bake for 25 minutes, or until the filling has set.
- Let the bars cool fully before sprinkling with powdered sugar.

Nutrition Facts:

- Calories: 300
- Carbohydrates: 40 grams
- Fat: 15 grams
- Protein: 5 grams
- Fiber: 2 grams

Tips

- For a gluten-free version, use gluten-free flour.

- For a dairy-free version, use dairy-free butter.
- For a vegan version, use a vegan egg replacement.
- If you don't have an air fryer, you may bake the bars in a preheated oven at 325 degrees F for 30-35 minutes, or until the filling is set.

3. Low FODMAP Chocolate Mousse

This recipe is for a tasty and easy-to-make Low FODMAP Chocolate Mousse. It is produced with only a few basic ingredients and may be cooked in an air fryer. The mousse is thick and creamy, and it is the ideal dessert for any occasion.

Preparation Time: 10 minutes
Cooking Time: 5 minutes
Total Time: 15 minutes

Ingredients:

- 1 cup (240ml) heavy cream
- 1/2 cup (100g) dark chocolate, chopped
- 1/4 cup (50g) sugar
- 1/4 cup (50g) cocoa powder
- 1/4 teaspoon salt

Instructions:

- In a medium bowl, mix the heavy cream, chocolate, sugar, cocoa powder, and salt.
- Microwave the mixture in 30-second increments, stirring in between, until the chocolate is melted and the liquid is smooth.
- Pour the mixture into an air fryer basket and cook at 350 degrees Fahrenheit for 5 minutes.
- Let the mousse cool for 10 minutes before serving.

Nutrition:

- Calories: 250
- Carbohydrates: 15g
- Fat: 15g
- Protein: 5g
- Fiber: 2g

Tips

- For a richer mousse, use dark chocolate with a greater cocoa content.
- For a more robust chocolate taste, add 1/4 teaspoon of espresso powder to the mixture.
- Serve the mousse immediately or refrigerate it for later.
- The mousse may be kept in the refrigerator for up to 3 days.

4. Low FODMAP Chocolate Chip Cookies

These low FODMAP chocolate chip cookies are prepared in the air fryer, which resulting in chewy, gooey cookies that are excellent for a fast and simple treat. The dish is also gluten-free and dairy-free, making it a wonderful alternative for anyone with dietary limitations.

Preparation time: 10 minutes
Cooking time: 10 minutes
Total time: 20 minutes

Ingredients:

- 1/2 cup (1 stick) unsalted butter, softened
- 1/2 cup brown sugar, packed
- 1/2 cup granulated sugar
- 2 eggs

- 1 teaspoon vanilla extract
- 1 1/2 cups gluten-free or ordinary all-purpose flour
- 1/2 teaspoon salt
- 1/2 teaspoon baking soda
- 1/2 teaspoon baking powder
- 1 cup chocolate chips

Instructions:

- Preheat the air fryer to 300 degrees Fahrenheit.
- In a large bowl, beat together the butter, brown sugar, and granulated sugar until light and fluffy.
- Beat in the eggs one at a time, then whisk in the vanilla essence.
- In a separate dish, mix together the flour, salt, baking soda, and baking powder.
- Gradually add the dry ingredients to the wet components, mixing until just incorporated.
- Stir in the chocolate chips.
- Drop the dough by rounded spoonful onto a parchment-lined air fryer basket.
- Cook for 8-10 minutes, or until the cookies are golden brown.
- Let cool on the parchment paper for a few minutes before transferring to a wire rack to cool fully.

Nutrition:

One cookie comprises approximately:

Calories: 150

Carbs: 20 grams

Fat: 8 grams

Protein: 2 grams

Fiber: 1 gram

Tips

- For chewier cookies, refrigerate the dough for at least 30 minutes before baking.
- To prevent the cookies from spreading too much, do not overmix the dough.
- If you don't have an air fryer, you may bake the cookies in a preheated oven at 350 degrees Fahrenheit for 10-12 minutes, or until golden brown.

5. Low FODMAP Popsicles

Low FODMAP popsicles are a delightful and refreshing dessert that is suitable for persons with irritable bowel syndrome (IBS) or other digestive disorders. They are produced with basic ingredients that are low in FODMAPs, a type of short-chain carbohydrates that may cause symptoms in persons with IBS.

Preparation Time: 10 minutes
Cooking Time: 20 minutes
Total Time: 30 minutes

Ingredients:

- 1 cup of frozen berries (any sort)
- 1/2 cup of milk (any sort)
- 1/2 cup of yogurt (any variety)
- 1 spoonful of honey
- 1/4 teaspoon of vanilla extract

Instructions:

In a blender, mix all of the ingredients.
- Puree till smooth.
- Pour the mixture into popsicle molds.

- Freeze for at least 20 minutes, or until solid.
- Enjoy!

Nutritional Information:

One low FODMAP popsicle produced with the components indicated above comprises approximately:

- Calories: 100
- Carbohydrates: 20 grams
- Fat: 1 gram
- Protein: 5 grams
- Fiber: 3 grams

Tips

- For a more savory popsicle, you may add a few drops of your favorite essential oil, such as peppermint or lemon.
- If you don't have an air fryer, you may freeze the popsicles in a standard freezer. However, it may take longer for them to freeze solid.
- You may also use other varieties of fruit in your popsicles. Some nice possibilities are strawberries, raspberries, blueberries, and mango.
- Get creative with your toppings! Some interesting possibilities include chocolate chips, shredded coconut, and crushed almonds.

6. Low FODMAP Fruit Salad

This Low FODMAP Fruit Salad is a tasty and nutritious way to enjoy a variety of fruits. The air fryer helps to caramelize the fruits and bring out their inherent sweetness. This salad is excellent for a light snack or dessert.

Preparation time: 10 minutes

Cooking time: 10-12 minutes

Total time: 20-22 minutes

Ingredients:

- 1 papaya, peeled and diced
- 1 pineapple, peeled, cored, and sliced
- 1 cantaloupe, peeled, seeded, and diced
- 2 cups red grapes
- 1 tablespoon honey
- 1/2 teaspoon ground cinnamon
- 1/4 teaspoon ground nutmeg

Instructions:

- Preheat the air fryer to 350 degrees F (175 degrees C).
- In a large bowl, mix the papaya, pineapple, cantaloupe, and grapes.
- In a small dish, mix the honey, cinnamon, and nutmeg.
- Pour the honey mixture over the fruit and toss to coat.
- Spread the fruit in a single layer in the air fryer basket.
- Air fry for 10-12 minutes, or until the fruit is soft and slightly browned.
- Serve immediately.

Nutrition:

- Calories: 180
- Carbohydrates: 35 grams
- Fat: 0 grams
- Protein: 3 grams
- Fiber: 10 grams

Tips

- For a more powerful taste, you may increase the quantity of honey or add additional spices such as cardamom or ginger.
- You may also use additional low FODMAP fruits in this salad, such as berries, kiwi, or mango.
- The fruit salad may be served warm or cold.

7. Low FODMAP Yogurt Parfait

This recipe is for a tasty and easy-to-make Low FODMAP Yogurt Parfait that can be cooked in an air fryer. The parfait is constructed with layers of yogurt, granola, and fruit, and it is a fantastic way to get your daily dosage of probiotics and fiber. The air fryer cooks the parfait evenly and gives it a lovely, crispy crust.

Preparation Time: 5 minutes
Cooking Time: 10-12 minutes
Total Time: 15-17 minutes

Ingredients:

- 1 cup of plain yogurt
- 1/2 cup of granola
- 1/2 cup of berries, such as blueberries, raspberries, or strawberries
- 1 spoonful of honey
- 1/4 teaspoon of cinnamon

Instructions:

- In a small bowl, mix the yogurt, granola, berries, honey, and cinnamon.
- Pour the ingredients into a ramekin or other small dish that is oven-safe.

- Cook the parfait in the air fryer at 350 degrees Fahrenheit for 10-12 minutes, or until the granola is golden brown and the yogurt is cooked through.
- Serve immediately and enjoy!

Nutrition Information:

- Calories: 250
- Carbohydrates: 30 grams
- Fat: 10 grams
- Protein: 10 grams
- Fiber: 5 grams

Tips

- For a more luxurious parfait, top with a scoop of whipped cream or a drizzle of chocolate sauce.
- If you don't have an air fryer, you may bake the parfait in a preheated oven at 350 degrees Fahrenheit for 15-20 minutes, or until the granola is golden brown and the yogurt is cooked through.
- This recipe is highly adapted to your personal tastes. You may use several kinds of yogurt, granola, and fruit. You may also add additional ingredients, such as almonds, seeds, or chocolate chips.

8. Low FODMAP Apples

These low FODMAP apples are a delightful and healthful snack or dessert. They are created with only a few basic ingredients and then baked in an air fryer for a crispy, caramelized finish.

Preparation time: 10 minutes
Cooking time: 10-12 minutes
Total time: 20-22 minutes

Ingredients:

- 2 apples, cored and sliced
- 1 tablespoon of lemon juice
- 1 teaspoon of ground cinnamon
- 1/2 teaspoon of ground nutmeg
- 1/4 teaspoon of salt
- 1 tablespoon of sugar

Instructions:

- Preheat the air fryer to 350 degrees Fahrenheit.
- In a large bowl, mix the apples, lemon juice, cinnamon, nutmeg, salt, and sugar.
- Toss to coat the apples evenly.
- Spread the apples in a single layer in the air fryer basket.
- Air fry for 10-12 minutes, or until the apples are soft and slightly caramelized.
- Serve heated or at room temperature.

Nutrition Information (per serving):

- Calories: 120
- Carbohydrates: 25 grams
- Fat: 0 grams
- Protein: 2 grams
- Fiber: 5 grams

Tips

- For a sweeter flavor, add an extra tablespoon of sugar.
- For a more tart flavor, reduce the amount of sugar to 1/2 tablespoon.

- To make the apples ahead of time, air fry them according to the instructions, then let them cool completely. Store them in an airtight container at room temperature for up to 2 days. To reheat, simply air fry them for an additional 2-3 minutes, or until heated through.

9. Low FODMAP Peaches

This is a quick and easy recipe for making delicious, low FODMAP peaches in an air fryer. The peaches are cooked until they are soft and slightly caramelized, and they are flavored with a simple syrup made with honey, lemon juice, and cinnamon. This recipe is perfect for a light dessert or snack.

Preparation time: 5 minutes
Cooking time: 10-12 minutes
Total time: 15-17 minutes

Ingredients:

- 4 medium peaches, halved and pitted
- 2 tablespoons honey
- 1 tablespoon lemon juice
- 1/2 teaspoon ground cinnamon

Instructions:

- In a small bowl, stir together the honey, lemon juice, and cinnamon.
- Place the peach halves in the air fryer basket. Drizzle with the honey mixture and toss to coat.
- Air fried at 350 degrees F for 10-12 minutes, or until the peaches are tender and slightly caramelized.
- Serve immediately.

Nutrition:

One serving of this dish comprises approximately:

- Calories: 100
- Carbohydrates: 20 grams
- Fat: 0 grams
- Protein: 1 gram
- Fiber: 3 grams

Tips

- For a more powerful cinnamon taste, add an additional 1/4 teaspoon of ground cinnamon to the honey mixture.
- If you don't have an air fryer, you may simply bake the peaches in a preheated oven at 350 degrees F for 15-20 minutes, or until they are soft and slightly caramelized.
- Serve the peaches warm or at room temperature.

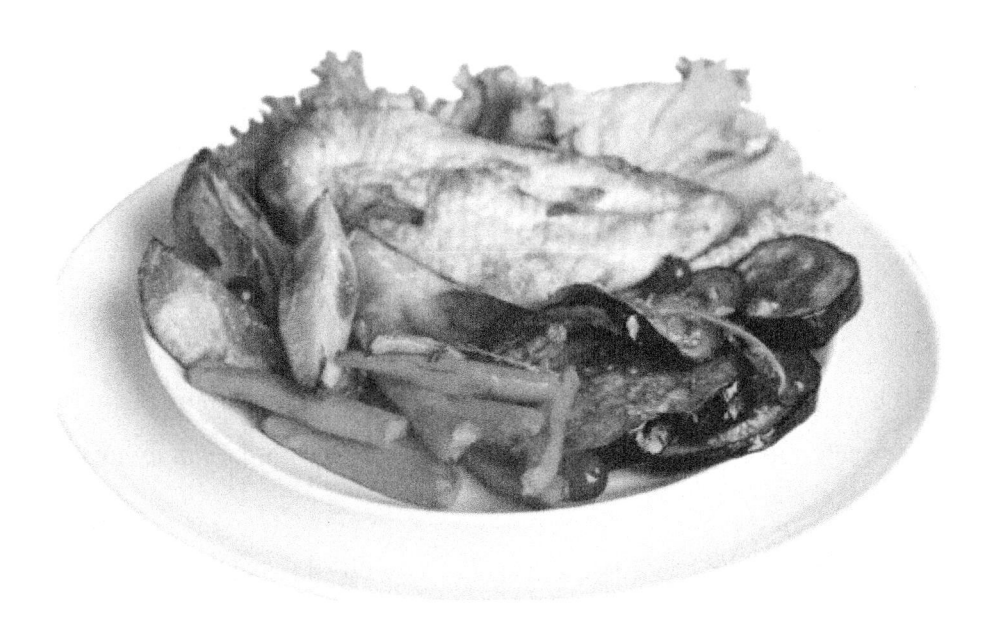

Chapter 8

Low Fodmap Air Fryer Snacks Recipes

1. Low FODMAP Guacamole and veggies

This dish is a terrific way to have a nutritious and tasty snack or supper. The guacamole is produced with low FODMAP components, so it is healthy for persons with irritable bowel syndrome (IBS) or other digestive diseases. The veggies are air fried to perfection, making them crunchy and delicious.

Preparation time: 10 minutes
Cooking time: 10-12 minutes
Total time: 20-22 minutes

Ingredients:

- 2 ripe avocados
- 1/2 onion, chopped 1 tomato, chopped
- 1/4 cup cilantro, chopped
- 1/4 teaspoon salt
- 1/4 teaspoon black pepper
- 1/4 cup vegetable oil
- 1 pound veggies, such as **carrots**, broccoli, or zucchini, chopped into bite-sized pieces

Instructions:

- To create the guacamole, mash the avocados in a bowl. Add the onion, tomato, cilantro, salt, and pepper. Stir to mix.

- To air fried the veggies, prepare the air fryer to 400 degrees Fahrenheit. Toss the veggies with the vegetable oil. Air fried for 10-12 minutes, or until soft and crispy.
- Serve the guacamole with the air fried veggies.

Nutrition:

- Calories: 250
- Carbohydrates: 15 grams
- Fat: 20 grams
- Protein: 5 grams
- Fiber: 5 grams

Tips

- For a hotter guacamole, add a jalapeño pepper, seeded and minced.
- For a smoother guacamole, use a food processor to mash the avocados.
- To air fry various veggies, just adjust the cooking time according to the kind of vegetable. For example, carrots will need to cook for a longer length of time than zucchini.

2. Low FODMAP Pizza Dough

Low FODMAP hash browns are a delightful and simple way to enjoy a staple breakfast item without any of the digestive pain. This dish is produced with only a few basic ingredients and may be cooked in an air fryer for a healthier choice than frying.

Preparation time: 10 minutes
Cooking time: 15-20 minutes
Total time: 25-30 minutes

Ingredients:

- 2 russet potatoes, peeled and grated
- 1 tablespoon olive oil
- 1/2 teaspoon salt
- 1/4 teaspoon black pepper

Instructions:

- Preheat the air fryer to 400 degrees Fahrenheit.
- In a large bowl, add the grated potatoes, olive oil, salt, and pepper.
- Toss to coat the potatoes evenly.
- Spread the potatoes in a single layer in the air fryer basket.
- Cook for 15-20 minutes, or until the potatoes are golden brown and crispy.
- Serve immediately.

Nutrition Information:

- Calories: 150
- Carbohydrates: 25 grams
- Fat: 10 grams
- Protein: 3 grams
- Fiber: 3 grams

Tips

- For extra crispy hash browns, preheat the oven to 400 degrees Fahrenheit and bake the hash browns for an additional 5-10 minutes after cooking in the air fryer.
- To prepare hash browns ahead of time, grate the potatoes and lay them in a basin. Toss with olive oil, salt, and pepper. Cover the bowl and chill for up to 24 hours. When you're ready to cook, preheat the air fryer and cook the hash browns according to the directions.

- Hash browns may be served with a number of toppings, such as ketchup, sour cream, or salsa.

3. Low FODMAP Quesadillas

Low FODMAP quesadillas are a tasty and simple way to enjoy a cheese, crunchy snack or supper. They are created using gluten-free tortillas, low FODMAP cheese, and your favorite toppings. Air frying the quesadillas gives them a crunchy top and a warm, gooey middle.

Preparation Time: 5 minutes
Cooking Time: 5-7 minutes
Total Time: 10-12 minutes

Ingredients:

- 2 gluten-free tortillas
- 1/2 cup low FODMAP cheese, shredded
- 1/4 cup diced onion
- 1/4 cup chopped bell pepper
- 1/4 cup diced tomato
- 1 tablespoon taco seasoning
- Salt and pepper to taste

Instructions:

- Preheat the air fryer to 350 degrees Fahrenheit.
- In a small bowl, mix the onion, bell pepper, tomato, taco seasoning, salt, and pepper.
- Spread half of the cheese on one tortilla. Top with the veggie mixture and the remaining cheese.
- Fold the tortilla in half and set it in the air fryer basket.
- Air fry for 5-7 minutes, or until the cheese is melted and the tortilla is golden brown.

- Repeat with the remaining tortilla.
- Cut the quesadillas into wedges and serve immediately.

Nutrition:

One quesadilla includes approximately:

- Calories: 200
- Carbohydrates: 25 grams
- Fat: 10 grams
- Protein: 10 grams
- Fiber: 5 grams

Tips

- Use your favorite low FODMAP toppings, such as cooked chicken, beans, or salsa.
- If you don't have an air fryer, you may cook these quesadillas in a pan on the stovetop. Just heat a pan over medium heat and cook the quesadillas for 2-3 minutes each side, or until the cheese is melted and the tortilla is golden brown.
- These quesadillas are a terrific entrée for lunch or supper. They are also an excellent alternative for gatherings or potlucks.

4. Low FODMAP Taquitos

Low FODMAP taquitos are a tasty and simple way to enjoy a Mexican-inspired lunch without having to worry about triggering your symptoms. Made with minimal ingredients, these taquitos can be fried in an air fryer for a fast and nutritious lunch.

Preparation Time: 15 minutes
Cooking Time: 10 minutes
Total Time: 25 minutes

Ingredients:

- 1 pound ground beef
- 1 onion, chopped
- 1 green bell pepper, chopped 1 (15 ounce) can black beans, drained and rinsed
- 1 (10 ounce) can corn, drained
- 1 cup shredded cheddar cheese
- 12 (6 inch) corn tortillas
- 1 tablespoon taco seasoning
- 1/4 cup olive oil

Instructions:

- Preheat your air fryer to 375 degrees F.
- In a large pan, cook the ground beef over medium heat. Drain off any excess oil.
- Add the onion and green pepper to the pan and simmer until softened, approximately 5 minutes.
- Stir in the black beans, corn, and taco seasoning. Cook for 1 minute more.
- Remove the pan from the heat and mix in the shredded cheese.
- To construct the taquitos, distribute approximately 1/2 cup of the meat mixture down the middle of each tortilla.
- Roll up the tortillas and fasten with toothpicks.
- Brush the taquitos with olive oil.
- Air fried the taquitos for 10 minutes, or until golden brown and crispy.
- Serve immediately.

Nutrition Information:

- Calories: 250
- Carbohydrates: 20 grams

- Fat: 15 grams
- Protein: 15 grams
- Fiber: 5 grams

Tips

- For a hotter taquitos, add a sprinkle of cayenne pepper to the ground beef mixture.
- You may also use ground chicken or turkey in this recipe.
- If you don't have an air fryer, you may bake the taquitos in a preheated oven at 400 degrees F for 15-20 minutes, or until golden brown and crispy.

5. Low FODMAP Pita Chips

These low FODMAP pita chips are a great and healthful snack or appetizer. They are baked using whole wheat pita bread, which is a healthy source of fiber. The air fryer approach guarantees that they are crispy and golden brown without being oily.

Preparation Time: 10 minutes
Cooking Time: 15 minutes
Total Time: 25 minutes

Ingredients:

- 2 whole wheat pita breads, cut into wedges
- 1 tablespoon olive oil
- 1/2 teaspoon salt
- 1/4 teaspoon black pepper

Instructions:

- Preheat the air fryer to 350 degrees Fahrenheit.

- In a small bowl, add the olive oil, salt, and pepper.
- Brush the pita wedges with the olive oil mixture.
- Air fried the pita wedges for 10-15 minutes, or until they are crispy and golden brown.
- Serve immediately.

Nutrition Facts:

- Calories: 120
- Carbohydrates: 20 grams
- Fat: 4 grams
- Protein: 3 grams
- Fiber: 4 grams

Tips

- For a more savory chip, you may add your favorite spices to the olive oil combination.
- If you don't have an air fryer, you may bake the pita chips in a preheated oven at 350 degrees Fahrenheit for 15-20 minutes, or until they are crispy and golden brown.
- These chips may be kept in an airtight container at room temperature for up to 3 days.

6. Low FODMAP Popcorn

This recipe for Low FODMAP Popcorn in an Air Fryer is a delightful and simple way to have a nutritious snack. The popcorn is manufactured with low FODMAP components, thus it is suitable for persons with irritable bowel syndrome (IBS). The air fryer process guarantees that the popcorn is light and fluffy, with a precise crunch.

Preparation Time: 5 minutes
Cooking Time: 10 minutes
Total Time: 15 minutes

Ingredients:

- 1/2 cup popcorn kernels
- 1 tablespoon olive oil
- 1/2 teaspoon salt
- 1/4 teaspoon garlic powder
- 1/4 teaspoon onion powder

Instructions:

- Preheat the air fryer to 350 degrees Fahrenheit.
- In a medium bowl, mix the popcorn kernels, olive oil, salt, garlic powder, and onion powder.
- Pour the popcorn mixture into the air fryer basket.
- Cook the popcorn for 10 minutes, or until it has popped and golden brown.
- Serve immediately.

Nutrition:

One serving of this dish (approximately 1 cup) includes the following nutrients:

- Calories: 120
- Carbohydrates: 17 grams
- Fat: 9 grams
- Protein: 3 grams
- Fiber: 2 grams

Tips

- If you do not have an air fryer, you may prepare this popcorn in a conventional oven. Preheat the oven to 350 degrees Fahrenheit and put the popcorn kernels on a baking sheet. Bake for 10 minutes, or until the popcorn has popped and golden brown.
- You may tweak the seasonings to your preference. For example, you may add more garlic powder and onion powder for a deeper taste, or you could add more paprika for a touch of spice.
- This popcorn is best eaten fresh, but it may also be kept in an airtight container at room temperature for up to 3 days.

7. Low FODMAP Celery with Peanut Butter

This dish is a fast and simple way to have a tasty and healthy snack. Celery is a low-FODMAP food, which means it is safe for persons with irritable bowel syndrome (IBS) to consume. Peanut butter is also a fantastic source of protein and fiber, which may assist to keep you feeling full and content. The air fryer cooks the celery and peanut butter combined, producing a crunchy and savory snack that is suitable for any time of day.

Preparation Time: 5 minutes
Cooking Time: 5-7 minutes
Total Time: 10-12 minutes

Ingredients:

- 1 bunch of celery, cleaned and sliced into sticks
- 1/4 cup peanut butter
- 1/4 teaspoon salt
- 1/8 teaspoon black pepper

Instructions:

- Preheat the air fryer to 350 degrees Fahrenheit.
- In a small bowl, mix the peanut butter, salt, and pepper.
- Toss the celery sticks in the peanut butter mixture until coated.
- Spread the celery sticks in a single layer in the air fryer basket.
- Air fry for 5-7 minutes, or until the celery is soft and the peanut butter is somewhat melted.
- Serve immediately and enjoy!

Nutrition Facts:

One serving of this dish comprises approximately:

- Calories: 150
- Carbohydrates: 15 grams
- Fat: 10 grams
- Protein: 5 grams
- Fiber: 4 grams

Tips

- For a more delicious snack, consider adding some chopped nuts or seeds to the peanut butter combination.
- If you don't have an air fryer, you may bake the celery sticks in a preheated oven at 350 degrees Fahrenheit for 10-12 minutes, or until they are soft.
- This dish is also a terrific way to use up leftover celery. Simply chop the celery and add it to the peanut butter mixture. Then, air fry or bake the celery sticks as recommended.

8. Low FODMAP Apples with Peanut Butter

This dish is a great and simple way to enjoy apples and peanut butter. The apples are fried in an air fryer until they are mushy and slightly caramelized, and then they are covered with peanut butter. This is a fantastic snack or dessert that is also low in FODMAPs.

Preparation Time: 10 minutes
Cooking Time: 10-12 minutes
Total Time: 20-22 minutes

Ingredients:

- 2 apples, peeled, cored, and sliced
- 1 tbsp peanut butter
- 1/4 teaspoon ground cinnamon

Instructions:

- Preheat the air fryer to 350 degrees Fahrenheit.
- In a medium bowl, combine together the apples, peanut butter, and cinnamon.
- Spread the apple mixture in a single layer in the air fryer basket.
- Air fried for 10-12 minutes, or until the apples are tender and slightly caramelized.
- Serve warm.

Nutrition:

- Calories: 150
- Carbohydrates: 25 grams
- Fat: 8 grams
- Protein: 5 grams
- Fiber: 5 grams

Tips

- For a sweeter snack, add a sprinkle of honey or maple syrup to the apples before serving.
- If you don't have an air fryer, you may bake the apples in a preheated oven at 350 degrees Fahrenheit for 15-20 minutes, or until they are soft and slightly caramelized.
- This dish is also gluten-free and vegan.

9. Low FODMAP Trail Mix

This recipe is for a tasty and nutritious Low FODMAP Trail Mix that can be cooked in an air fryer. The air fryer helps to crisp up the nuts and seeds, giving the trail mix a pleasant crunch. The trail mix is also a wonderful source of protein, fiber, and healthy fats.

Preparation time: 10 minutes
Cooking time: 10-12 minutes
Total time: 20-22 minutes

Ingredients:

- 1 cup raw peanuts
- 1/2 cup almonds
- 1/4 cup cashews
- 1/4 cup raisins
- 1/4 cup dried cranberries
- 1 tablespoon pumpkin seeds
- 1 tablespoon sunflower seeds
- 1/2 teaspoon salt

Instructions:

- Preheat the air fryer to 350 degrees Fahrenheit.
- In a large bowl, mix all of the ingredients.
- Spread the trail mix in a single layer in the air fryer basket.
- Air fry for 10-12 minutes, or until the nuts and seeds are golden brown and aromatic.
- Let cool fully before serving.

Nutrition (per 1/2 cup serving):

- Calories: 200
- Carbohydrates: 15 grams
- Fat: 12 grams
- Protein: 6 grams
- Fiber: 5 grams

Tips

- Feel free to add additional components to your trail mix, such as dried fruit, chocolate chips, or other nuts.
- If you don't have an air fryer, you may bake the trail mix in a preheated oven at 350 degrees Fahrenheit for 15-20 minutes, or until the nuts and seeds are golden brown and aromatic.
- Store the trail mix in an airtight jar at room temperature for up to 1 week.

Conclusion

The Low FODMAP Air Fryer Cookbook is a great resource for people with digestive disorders who are looking for delicious and easy-to-make recipes. The book includes a wide variety of recipes, from appetizers to main courses to desserts, all of which are low in FODMAPs.

FODMAPs are short-chain carbohydrates that can trigger symptoms in people with digestive disorders, such as irritable bowel syndrome (IBS). By following the recipes in this book, people with digestive disorders can reduce their symptoms and improve their overall quality of life.

Here are some tips for people with digestive disorders who are looking to reduce their symptoms:

- **Follow a low FODMAP diet.** This means avoiding foods that are high in FODMAPs. The Low FODMAP Air Fryer Cookbook is a great resource for finding low FODMAP recipes.
- **Keep a food diary.** This can help you identify foods that trigger your symptoms. Once you know which foods trigger your symptoms, you can avoid them.
- **Manage stress.** Stress can worsen digestive symptoms. Find healthy ways to manage stress, such as exercise, yoga, or meditation.
- **Get enough sleep.** When you're well-rested, your digestive system can function better. Aim for 7-8 hours of sleep per night.
- **See a doctor.** If your digestive symptoms are severe or don't improve with diet and lifestyle changes, see a doctor. There may be an underlying medical condition that needs to be treated.

Following these tips can help people with digestive disorders reduce their symptoms and improve their overall quality of life.

Here are some additional advice for people with chronic digestive disorders:

- **Be patient.** It can take time to find a diet and lifestyle that work for you. Don't get discouraged if you don't see results immediately.
- **Be flexible.** You may need to make adjustments to your diet and lifestyle as your symptoms change.
- **Don't give up.** There are many things you can do to improve your digestive health. With patience and perseverance, you can find relief from your symptoms.

There is no further information.

Thank you for ordering this **"Low FODMAP Air Fryer Cookbook For Beginners"** and I hope that you like it.

If you have an experience with the book that you would want to share with me, I would highly appreciate it!

Please take a minute to write me a favorable review on the site on which you bought the book or any other online review community. By providing me the chance to gather feedback from you, you will assist to make this book better for future readers and help to broaden its reach.

When you finish your review, please add any comments on how I may improve this book. I am continuously working to make it the best that it can be for my readers.

To show my appreciation, I am offering a complimentary email consultation to answer any questions you may have about this book. Maybe you're confused on a certain concept or require help understanding it better - I'm here to help.

To take advantage of this offer, just drop me an email at jhendersonanne@gmail.com with the title "Book Consultation" and a brief description of whatever issue you need help with. I will do my best to get back to you within 24 hours with a useful response.

Don't forget to post a review on this book.

Thank you for making this purchase and I look forward to your email.

Suggestion For You!

Would you like to try another recipe made with DUTCH OVEN OR CAST IRON SKILLET? I have a comprehensive beginners guide on making different kinds of recipes with Dutch oven and Cast Iron Skillet.

- For Dutch Oven Click here here to access this book
- For Cast Iron Click here to access this book

Follow the link for the Kindle version while for the paperback version, you should just type the link on your "BROWSER" to Access It.

Thank you Once Again!

Printed in Great Britain
by Amazon